D0765113

The Comfort of Home® for Chronic Liver Disease

A Guide for Caregivers

The Comfort of Home® Caregiver book series is written for family and paraprofessional home caregivers who face the responsibilities of caring for aging friends, family, or clients. The disease-specific editions, often in collaboration with organizations supporting those conditions, address caregivers assisting people with those diseases.

Other Caregiver Resources from CareTrust Publications:

La comodidad del hogar® *(Spanish Edition)*
The Comfort of Home®: *A Complete Guide for Caregivers*
The Comfort of Home® *for Chronic Lung Disease*
The Comfort of Home® *for Chronic Heart Failure*
The Comfort of Home® *for Alzheimer's Disease*
The Comfort of Home® *Multiple Sclerosis Edition*
The Comfort of Home® *for Parkinson Disease*
The Comfort of Home® *for Stroke*
The Comfort of Home® *Caregiving Journal*
Caring in The Comfort of Home® *UK Edition*
The Comfort of Home® *Caregivers—Let's Take Care of You!* Meditation CD

Newsletters:

The Comfort of Home® *Caregiver Assistance News*
The Comfort of Home® *Grand-Parenting News*
The Comfort of Home® *Caregivers—Let's Take Care of You!*

Visit *www.comfortofhome.com* for forthcoming editions and other caregiver resources.

The Comfort of Home®

of Home®

for Chronic Liver Disease

A Guide for Caregivers

Maria M. Meyer and Paula Derr, RN

with

Lucy Mathew, NP and Jill Chang, PA-C

CareTrust Publications LLC

"Caring for you... caring for others."

Portland, Oregon

The Comfort of Home® for Chronic Liver Disease: A Guide for Caregivers

Published by: CareTrust Publications LLC
P.O. Box 10283
Portland, Oregon 97296-0283
(800) 565-1533
Fax (503) 221-7019

Publisher's Cataloging-in-Publication
(Provided by Quality Books, Inc.)

Meyer, Maria M., 1948-
    The comfort of home for chronic liver disease :
a guide for caregivers / Maria M. Meyer and Paula Derr ;
with Lucy Mathew and Jill Chang.
        p. cm.
        Includes index.
        ISBN-13: 978-0-9787903-2-5
        ISBN-10: 0-9787903-2-4

    1. Home care services—Handbooks, manuals, etc.
2. Caregivers—Handbooks, manuals, etc. 3. Liver—
Diseases. 4. Chronic diseases.   I. Derr, Paula.
II. Title.

RA645.3.M4938 2008   649.8
                                      QBI08-854

Cover Art and Text Illustration: Stacey L. Tandberg
Interior Design: Frank Loose
Cover Design: David Kessler
Page Layout: Lapiz

Distributed to the Trade by Publishers Group West.
Printed in the United States of America.

08 09 10 11 12/10 9 8 7 6 5 4 3 2 1

About the Authors

Maria M. Meyer has been a long-time advocate of social causes, beginning with her work as co-founder of the Society for Abused Children of the Children's Home Society of Florida and founding executive director of the Children's Foundation of Greater Miami. When her father-in-law suffered a stroke in 1993, Maria became aware of the need for better information about how to care for an aging parent, a responsibility shared by millions of Americans. That experience led Maria to found CareTrust Publications and to co-author the award-winning guide, *The Comfort of Home®: An Illustrated Step-by-Step Guide for Caregivers*—now in its third edition. This book earned the Benjamin Franklin Award in the health category, as well as *Finalist* in ForeWord Magazine's 2007 Book of the Year Award. She is a keynote speaker and workshop leader on caregiver topics to health care professionals and community groups, as well as a Caregiver Community Action Network volunteer for the National Family Caregiver Association.

Paula Derr, RN, BSN, CEN, CCRN, has been employed by the Sisters of Providence Health System for over 30 years. She has broad experience in many different clinical settings and for many years served as clinical educator for three emergency departments in the Portland metropolitan area. She was a founder of inforMed, which publishes emergency medical services field guides for emergency medical technicians (EMTs), paramedics, firefighters, physicians, and nurses and has co-authored numerous health care articles. For Paula, home care is a family tradition of long standing. For many years, Paula cared for her mother and grandmother in her home while raising two daughters and maintaining her career in nursing and health care management. Her personal and professional experience adds depth to many chapters of this book. Paula is active in several prominent professional organizations and has held both local and national board positions. Paula is a native Oregonian and lives with her husband in Portland.

Lucy Mathew, NP is a nationally certified Nurse Practitioner with a Masters degree in the specialty of Acute Care Nurse Practitioner from UCLA. She has nine years of experience as a Nurse Practitioner. For the past five years, she has been managing patients with hepatitis B, hepatitis C, cirrhosis, and post transplant patients. She has medically managed pre- and post-operative cardiac surgery patients. She also has six years of experience in medical/surgical and critical care units as a registered nurse. Lucy works in Los Angeles at the Cedars Sinai Medical Center liver transplant department. She is actively involved in teaching other health care members about the importance of recognizing liver disease early and preventing complications. She is passionate about the subject and takes an active role in teaching physicians, nurses, and the community about liver disease.

Jill Chang, **PA-C** is a nationally certified Physician Assistant in the field of Hepatology and liver transplantation. For the past 2 years, she has been managing patients with chronic liver disease including pre- and post-liver transplant patients. She has worked in general Gastroenterology with special emphasis in Hepatology. She works in Los Angeles at Cedars-Sinai Medical Center liver transplant department and teaches Physician Assistant students as a guest lecturer at the University of Southern California Physician Assistant program. Jill is passionate about the field of hepatology and is proactive in community outreach activities in teaching the transmission and prevention of the various liver diseases.

Our Mission

CareTrust Publications is committed to providing high-quality, user-friendly information to those who face an illness or the responsibilities of caring for friends, family, or clients.

Dedication

We dedicate this book to Dr. Fred Poordad, Dr. Tram Tran, and Dr. Julie Winn for teaching us everything we know about liver disease. We give special thanks to them for their continuous support, constant encouragement, and their belief in our abilities.

—Lucy Mathew and Jill Chang

Dear Caregiver,

When a family member is diagnosed with chronic liver disease, you, the caregiver, will have to know and understand how the disease needs to be treated and what level of care is required.

The Comfort of Home® for Chronic Liver Disease: A Guide for Caregivers is a basic, complete guide that will answer your questions about caregiving. Covering current best practices for home care, it offers practical tips for everyday problems as well as more complicated and stressful situations, such as waiting for a liver transplant.

The *Guide* is divided into three parts:

Part One, **Getting Ready**, describes the types of chronic liver disease and how the disease affects the person in your care. You will learn how to choose a good medical team, keep costs down, and get the best, least expensive medicines. There is information about making the home safe and comfortable, paying for care and how to make important decisions about the future.

Part Two, **Day-by-Day** tells you how to develop a daily schedule and understand the challenges of living with chronic liver disease, its special care needs, such as getting proper nutrition and recognizing emergencies, and when to call an ambulance.

Part Three, **Additional Resources**, provides a glossary of common medical terms to help you understand the language that many health care professionals use to talk about liver disease. It also includes a list of references for further reading and information about organizations and publications for caregivers.

Armed with knowledge, you will feel confident that you can provide good care. With this *Guide* in hand, you will understand what help is needed and learn where to find it or how to provide it yourself.

Warm regards,

Maria, Paula, Lucy & Jill

Acknowledgments

The information in this *Guide* is based on research and consultation with experts in the fields of nursing, medicine, and design. The authors thank the innumerable professionals and caregivers who have assisted in the development of this book.

We thank Steven Chen, MD and Mathai Valumathahil whose critique, suggestions and edits were invaluable to this project. We also give special thanks to Dr. Andrew Klein, Director of the Comprehensive Transplant Center, Cedars Sinai Medical Center, for referring us to this project which will support the caregivers of liver disease patients.

This volume would not have been possible without the guidance, reviews and support of the following professionals at Cedars Sinai Medical Center in Los Angeles, California:

Fred Poordad, MD
Chief of Hepatology and Liver Transplant
Cedars Sinai Medical Center

Tram Tran, MD
Medical Director of Hepatology and Liver Transplant
Cedars Sinai Medical Center

Julie Winn, MD
Assistant Medical Director of Hepatology and Liver Transplant
Cedars Sinai Medial Center

Some sections of this volume are adapted from other editions in the *Comfort of Home®* series. We extend our gratitude to those authors and organizations whose contributions have also enhanced this edition.

To Our Readers

We believe *The Comfort of Home® for Chronic Liver Disease: A Guide for Caregivers* reflects currently accepted practice in the areas it covers. However, the authors and publisher assume no liability with respect to the accuracy, completeness, or application of information presented here.

The Comfort of Home® for Chronic Liver Disease is not meant to replace medical care but to add to the medical advice and services you receive from health care professionals. You should seek professional medical advice from a health care provider. This book is only a guide; follow your common sense and good judgment.

Neither the authors nor the publisher are engaged in rendering legal, accounting, or other professional advice. Seek the services of a competent professional if legal, architectural, or other expert assistance is required. The *Guide* does not represent Americans with Disabilities Act compliance.

Every effort has been made at the time of publication to provide accurate names, addresses, and phone numbers in the resource sections at the ends of chapters. The resources listed are those that benefit readers nationally. For this reason we have not included many local groups that offer valuable assistance. Failure to include an organization does not mean that it does not provide a valuable service. On the other hand, inclusion does not imply an endorsement. The authors and publisher do not warrant or guarantee any of the products described in this book and did not perform any independent analysis of the products described.

Throughout the book, we use "he" and "she" interchangeably when referring to the caregiver and the person being cared for.

ATTENTION NONPROFIT ORGANIZATIONS, CORPORATIONS, AND PROFESSIONAL ORGANIZATIONS: *The Comfort of Home® for Chronic Liver Disease* is available at special quantity discounts for bulk purchases for gifts, fundraising, or educational training purposes. Special books, book excerpts, or booklets can also be created to fit specific needs. For details, write to CareTrust Publications LLC, P.O. Box 10283, Portland, Oregon 97296-0283, or call 1-800-565-1533.

✦ CONTENTS AT A GLANCE

Part Three   *Additional Resources*

CHAPTER

Praise for *The Comfort of Home*® Caregiver Guides

"This is an invaluable addition to bibliographies for the home caregiver. Hospital libraries will want to have a copy on hand for physicians, nurses, social workers, chaplains, and any staff dealing with MS patients and their caregivers. Highly recommended for all public libraries and consumer health collections."
—*Library Journal*

"A well-organized format with critical information and resources at your fingertips . . . educates the reader about the many issues that stand before people living with chronic conditions and provides answers and avenues for getting the best care possible."
—MSWorld, Inc. www.msworld.org

"A masterful job of presenting the multiple aspects of caregiving in a format that is both comprehensive and reader-friendly . . . important focus on physical aspects of giving care."
—Parkinson Report

"Almost any issue or question or need for resolution is most likely spoken of somewhere within the pages of this guide."
—*American Journal of Alzheimer's Disease*

"Physicians, family practitioners and geriatricians, and hospital social workers should be familiar with the book and recommend it to families of the elderly."
—Reviewers Choice, Home Care University

"An excellent guide on caregiving in the home. Home health professionals will find it to be a useful tool in teaching family caregivers."
—Five Star Rating, *Doody's Health Sciences Review Journal*

"Overall a beautifully designed book with very useful, practical information for caregivers."
—Judges from the Benjamin Franklin Awards

"Noteable here are the specifics. Where others focus on psychology alone, this gets down to the nitty gritty."
—*The Midwest Book Review*

"We use *The Comfort of Home*® for the foundational text in our 40-hour Caregiver training. I believe it is the best on the market."
—Linda Young, Project Manager, College of the Desert

Part One: Getting Ready

Understanding Liver Disease

Understanding Liver Disease

*W*hen a family member is diagnosed with chronic liver disease, you, the caregiver, will have to know and understand how the disease needs to be treated and what level of care is required. The level of care needed for someone with end-stage liver disease varies. The job can be as simple as making sure that the person follows up with the doctor, is on time for his appointments, helps the person in care make decisions, offer psychological support, etc. Or it can be as involved as giving physical care such as assisting with bathing, walking, etc.

Another example of care needed would be to closely watch or monitor the person's daily salt intake to avoid edema (swelling). Also you may need to titrate (measure) lactulose (a type of sugar that acts as a laxative) depending on his bowel movements and mental status (ability to think clearly).

When you become a caregiver, you may feel guilt, anger, fear that you are unable to do the job, or that you are a victim. At times you may feel constantly stressed. In order to survive, you will have to set limits and you will have to enforce rules, neither of which is comfortable. If you don't set limits and enforce rules, however, your life will become unmanageable, and the person you're caring for will suffer.

Part of reducing the stress you feel is to understand the condition and the effects it will have on the lifestyle of both you and the person in your care. It is also important to know from the beginning that you have to find ways to take care of yourself. Maybe fit a walk in while the person in your care is napping, or do 10 minutes of yoga after he goes to bed. Whatever it is, do something for yourself every day, even if it is just for a short time.

Here we give you a quick look at what to expect with each chronic liver condition. Your health care provider will explain *in more detail the particulars of the diagnosis (medical condition) of the person in your care and his particular care needs.*

What Is Liver Disease?

The liver is the largest internal solid organ in the human body. It is located on the right side of the abdomen, just under the rib cage. It helps with digestion, blood clotting, and control of blood glucose (sugar level in the blood). It stores vitamins and minerals. Its major job is the removal of toxic (poisonous) substances and detoxification (cleansing) of poisonous substances, such as alcohol, from the body. Think of the liver as a filter for all the good and bad things we eat and drink.

Most liver diseases do not have any symptoms, but can lead to cirrhosis (hardening of the liver from scar tissue) and liver failure if not treated properly. Because the liver has an amazing ability to regenerate (regrow), it can withstand injuries or abuse from an unhealthy lifestyle for many years, sometimes even decades. The good news is, if found early, most diseases can be controlled to prevent significant liver damage. Some liver diseases are contagious, some are hereditary (passed on genetically). Therefore it is important for the caregiver to be aware of the liver diagnosis. You, as caregiver should make sure that you are tested for any hereditary liver disease if you are related to the patient. You should make sure that the person in your care follows the appropriate steps to take care of himself.

Tip

Look through the list on the following pages to identify the diagnosis of liver disease. Read the details about it so that you have a better understanding of the disease.

Common Causes of Liver Disease

When you and the person in your care are with his health care provider you may hear terms you never heard before regarding the liver. The most common liver diseases are—

Viral Hepatitis

There are six different known viruses that can cause liver injury. They are hepatitis A, B, C, D, E, and G. Hepatitis A, B, and C are the most common. Hepatitis A is caused by drinking water and eating food that is contaminated with the virus. Recent outbreaks of hepatitis A were caused when people ate raw scallions infected with the virus. Once they have caught this virus, people can become ill with abdominal pain, nausea, vomiting, jaundice (yellowing of the skin), decreased appetite, and dark urine. These symptoms can last a few weeks to a few months. Fortunately, hepatitis A does not cause lifelong disease, but can recur up to one year after infection. The chance of complete liver failure requiring liver transplant in hepatitis A is less than 1% in healthy adults. People usually recover from hepatitis A and will develop lifelong immunity (they won't be able to get sick from hepatitis A again). Hepatitis B and C are much more serious infections and will be discussed in more detail later. (See **Hepatitis B and Hepatitis C,** page 13.)

> **NOTE** There is a safe Hepatitis A vaccination available for people over the age of two. It is given as a series of two shots, six months apart. The vaccine is recommended for anyone with liver disease and the caregiver should also receive the vaccine to prevent getting the infection.

Fatty Liver/NASH

Fatty liver is an accumulation of fat in the liver. Some people can have simple fat in the liver that may be harmless. However, fat can sometimes cause inflammation (swelling) and this is called nonalcoholic steatohepatitis (NASH). This can lead to scar tissue replacing the healthy liver tissue, which is known as cirrhosis, and eventually leads to liver failure. Fatty liver is a growing problem in this country as the population becomes overweight. The prevalence of fatty liver is 20 percent in the United States, whereas the prevalence of NASH is less than 10 percent. Fatty liver is caused by obesity, starvation, diabetes, certain medications, and drinking alcohol. The treatment is to change the underlying cause, such as losing weight if the cause is obesity.

Hemochromatosis

This is an inherited disorder (passed on from parents to children) that causes too much iron to be stored in the body. People with this disorder absorb too much iron from their food. Over many years this excess iron builds up in the organs and causes damage that can lead to disease, such as cirrhosis of the liver. About one out of 200 people in the United States have this problem. Lifelong treatment is needed to remove the excess iron from the liver through medication (chelation) or by removing blood (phlebotomy) from the body.

NOTE Because this is an inherited disorder, all first-degree relatives (parents and children, brothers and sisters) should get checked for this disease by doing simple blood tests.

Alpha-1-Antitrypsin Deficiency (AAT)

This is an inherited disorder that causes low levels or a complete lack of AAT in the blood. AAT is an enzyme made by the liver that is released into the bloodstream. AAT mainly protects the lungs from a harmful enzyme (neutrophil elastase). AAT deficiency is a disorder often overlooked by doctors that affects the lungs, liver, and rarely—the skin. Although AAT deficiency is considered to be rare, about 80,000 to 100,000 individuals in the United States have severe deficiency of AAT. Liver disorders, such as neonatal hepatitis (liver inflammation occurring just after birth), cirrhosis both in children and adults, and liver cancer are associated with some AAT deficiencies. Treatment options are very limited. Liver transplantation remains the only treatment for liver AAT disease.

 NOTE Because this is also an inherited disorder, all first-degree relatives should be checked.

Alcoholic Liver Disease

Alcoholic liver disease ranges from fatty liver, alcoholic hepatitis, to end-stage liver failure. Unfortunately, many alcoholics notice the first symptoms only when severe, life-threatening liver disease is already present. Alcohol-related chronic liver disease accounts for more than 12,000 deaths per year in the United States.

The best treatment for alcoholic liver disease is to abstain from alcohol. Even people with advanced liver disease caused by drinking alcohol can significantly improve the disease if they stop drinking. Abstinence (not drinking alcohol) is also critical for those patients with advanced disease who may eventually require liver transplantation. Transplant centers generally require that a person has not been drinking for at least 6 months to be eligible for transplant. Referral to an in-patient rehabilitation program or an Alcoholics Anonymous program is usually necessary in combination with family support and counseling. Continuing to drink alcohol is the single most important risk factor for worsening the condition.

Drug-Induced Liver Injury

This type of liver disease is caused by several medications and can result in inflammation of the liver and even liver failure. Liver toxicity (poisoning) caused by medication is the most common reason for acute liver failure in the United States. Medicines that can cause acute liver failure are chlorpromazine, sulfa drugs, birth control pills, acetaminophen (Tylenol), isoniazid, methyldopa, phenytoin, and aspirin. Medications called non-steroidal anti-inflammatory drugs (NSAIDS), which include Advil, Motrin, Ibuprofen, etc. can also cause injury to the liver—even liver failure if taken in sufficient doses.

NOTE Tylenol is known to be toxic to the liver at high doses. However, it is important to understand that it only causes liver failure when more than the *recommended daily dose* is taken. Tylenol is considered safe, even in patients with liver disease, as long as it is taken only as directed and in appropriate doses.

Wilson Disease

This is a rare disorder in which excess copper builds up in the body, affecting the liver, brain, and/or eyes. In the U. S., one in 30,000 individuals has this illness. People with Wilson disease can develop hepatitis or even liver failure in their early teens to mid-fifties. Neurological or psychiatric problems can also be symptoms of Wilson disease. Removal of copper using medication (chelation), if diagnosed early, is an effective treatment. However, liver transplant is necessary with liver failure.

Autoimmune Hepatitis (AIH)

Autoimmune hepatitis is a disease in which the body's immune system attacks the liver cells and causes inflammation, scar tissue, and cirrhosis. Symptoms can range from being asymptomatic (without symptoms) to severe jaundice, itching, abdominal pain, nausea, vomiting, decreased appetite, and fatigue. Effective treatments include steroids and immuno-suppressants (medication that stops the immune system from attacking). Autoimmune hepatitis can lead to liver failure over time if not treated properly.

NOTE About 70 percent of those with AIH are women between the ages of 15 and 40.

Primary Sclerosing Cholangitis (PSC)

PSC is a disease that most commonly affects young men. The disease is characterized by progressive inflammation and narrowing of medium and large bile ducts (bile ducts are small tubes in the liver that drain bile out of the liver into the gallbladder and small intestine). The prevalence of PSC in the general population is not known. People with PSC often have no symptoms at the time of diagnosis and many may already have had significant liver damage. Liver transplantation is now the treatment of choice for those with advanced PSC, and the five-year survival rate after transplantation is as high as 85 percent. Average survival without liver transplantation after diagnosis is approximately 12 years.

Primary Biliary Cirrhosis (PBC)

PBC is an autoimmune disorder that mainly affects women. It involves progressive destruction of small bile ducts, preventing drainage of bile from the liver. This bile accumulation in the liver can result in cirrhosis and liver failure. PBC very rarely occurs in childhood or before age 30. The onset is usually between the ages of 30 to 65. Unfortunately, the incidence of PBC is rising and the cause is unclear. Fatigue and itching are the most common symptoms of PBC, but half of people feel no symptoms. People with PBC do not absorb certain fat-soluble vitamins, A, D, E, K (vitamins stored in fat). Some of those individuals may be at increased risk for osteoporosis (bone thinning) due to vitamin D deficiency. These people should be evaluated and treated for osteoporosis.

Treatment of PBC is ursodeoxycholic acid, which is a pill that thins out the bile, and is well tolerated. It can often delay disease progression. Many people with early-stage PBC may have a normal life expectancy with treatment.

Find out more information about any of these liver disease conditions from the websites listed in the Resources or from your health care provider.

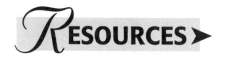

RESOURCES ➤

Alcoholics Anonymous
http://www.alcoholics-anonymous.org

American Liver Foundation
75 Maiden Lane Suite 603
New York, NY 10038
(212) 668-1000 Fax: (212) 483-8179
www.liverfoundation.org
The American Liver Foundation offers information and support to the 30 million Americans affected by liver disease.

Primary Sclerosing Cholangitis (PSC) Foundation
50 N Dunlap WPT
401 Memphis, TN 38103
(901) 287-5355
Pscfoundation.org
The PSC Foundation sponsors research to treat this disorder. The website offers information and support to patients and families.

The American Association for the Study of Liver Diseases (AASLD)
1001 North Fairfax, Suite 400
Alexandria, VA 22314
(703) 299-9766
Fax: (703) 299-9622
Email:aasld@aasld.org
www.aasld.org
Provides the public with information on how to contact a hepatologist.

The Hepatitis B Foundation
www.hepB.org
Information and resources for patients regarding treatment, programs and studies.

Hepatitis Central
www.hepatitis-central.com
Source for information on published articles, testing and treatment of hepatitis.

Hepatitis Foundation International On-line
www.hepfi.org
Provides education about viral hepatitis, prevention, diagnosis and treatment.

HIV and Hepatitis.com
www.hivandhepatitis.com
Information about treatment options for hepatitis A, B and C.

Hepatitis B and Hepatitis C

Hepatitis B and Hepatitis C

Hepatitis B

What Is It?

Liver disease can be caused by the hepatitis B virus (HBV). Most people who become infected with HBV are able to get rid of the virus from their bloodstream and develop immunity (resistance to the disease). Those who do not clear the virus after six months are considered to have chronic hepatitis B. However, not all patients with chronic hepatitis B will need treatment, and it is important that these people go to a specialist such as a gastroenterologist (stomach and intestine doctor) or a hepatologist (liver doctor) to find out whether or not they need treatment. Approximately 15 to 25 percent of the people chronically infected with hepatitis B will eventually die from liver disease.

Worldwide, chronic hepatitis B is the leading cause of liver cancer and is the sixth leading cause of liver transplantation. It is estimated that 1.25 million people have chronic hepatitis B in the United States, with the highest frequency in Asian Americans. As many as one out of 10 Asian Americans is infected with hepatitis B. Liver cancer due to hepatitis B is a leading cause of death for Vietnamese and Cambodian men. Asian Americans should be screened for hepatitis B and vaccinated if the test shows no immunity.

 If the person in your care has hepatitis B, make sure *you* are tested and vaccinated for hepatitis B. This is extremely important to prevent infection.

What Caregivers Need to Know

Hepatitis B virus can live outside the body for up to seven days. It can be found in blood, sperm, vaginal secretions, and saliva. HBV can be transmitted through—

- direct blood-to-blood contact

- vertical transmission (from an infected mother to her baby during/around childbirth)

- unprotected sex

- intimate kissing

- unsterile needles

- tattooing, body piercing, or acupuncture with infected needles

- sharing razors, toothbrushes, earrings, or other personal items that may come in contact with blood

The virus is rarely found in tears, urine, feces, sweat, and breast milk, therefore it is considered to be safe for mothers with hepatitis B to breastfeed without serious risk of passing the disease to their babies, provided the baby is vaccinated.

Acute infection (serious sudden infection) with hepatitis B virus is an illness that begins with fatigue, loss of appetite, abdominal pain, nausea, vomiting, body aches, mild fever, dark urine, and may then progress to the development of jaundice (yellowish eyes and skin). Itchy skin is common. The acute infection may also occur entirely without symptoms and often goes unrecognized. In most people, the illness lasts for a few weeks and then gradually gets better. A few people may have more severe liver disease, including liver failure and may die as a result of it.

Chronic infection (constant infection) with hepatitis B virus may be without symptoms. It can be an inflammation of the liver that does not go away—even leading to cirrhosis (scarring of the liver) over a period of years.

> **NOTE** ▶ All chronic hepatitis B patients are at risk for developing liver cancer even when they have no scar tissue or other signs of liver disease, so it is important for these people to be checked for liver cancer at least once a year. If a person with hepatitis B has liver failure or liver cancer, then liver transplant is the best treatment.

To find out if a person has hepatitis B he or she needs to have a set of simple blood tests. All people at risk should be tested, including—

- all immigrants from areas of high prevalence (Asia, Africa, etc.)

- people with multiple sex partners or history of a sexually transmitted disease

- men who have sex with men

- people who have sex with people who have hepatitis B

- injection drug users

- household contacts with chronically infected people

- infants born to infected mothers

- infants/children of immigrants from areas with high rates of HBV infection (i.e., Asia, Africa)

- health care and public safety workers

- dialysis patients

All people at risk who do not have hepatitis B should get the vaccine for hepatitis B. This vaccine consists of three shots given over a period of six months. These shots are now part of the routine set of vaccinations for all people between 0 and 18 years old. Since the discovery of the vaccine, hepatitis B has gone down significantly. The vaccine is very safe.

Hepatitis B is not a curable disease. The goal of treatment is to keep the virus from replicating (reproducing) and hopefully reduce the complications associated with the virus, such as liver cirrhosis (scarring), liver failure, and liver cancer.

Here is a list of medicines available to treat hepatitis B:

- Interferon/ pegylated interferon alpha-2a (immune system modulators)

- Lamivudine (Epivir)

- Adefovir (Hepsera)

- Entecavir (Baraclude)

- Telbivudine (Tyzeka)

 Some of these medications are injections and the caregiver may have to give these injections to the patient.

Remember, not all people with hepatitis B need treatment. It is important for them to go to a specialist to see if they need treatment and, if so, which treatment is best for them.

Hepatitis C

What Is It?

Hepatitis C (HCV) is a virus that gets into the body through the blood and attacks the liver. Most people get hepatitis C by coming in contact with contaminated blood. HCV can be transmitted through:

- injection drug use

- snorting drugs

- tattoos

- blood transfusion prior to 1992

- vertical transmission (mother to baby)

- sexual relationships with blood exposure

 People from Egypt should be screened for hepatitis C due to high infection rates.

What the Caregiver Needs to Know

Hepatitis C usually has no symptoms. It can lead to swelling and scar tissue forming in the liver. Some people can develop cirrhosis (liver scar tissue), but it usually takes 20–30 years to develop cirrhosis. Once cirrhosis sets in, people are at risk for developing liver cancer and liver failure. Unlike hepatitis B, where cancer can occur without cirrhosis, liver cancer due to hepatitis C almost always develops after cirrhosis or advanced fibrosis formation.

 Seventy-five percent of people who are infected with hepatitis C virus eventually develop chronic hepatitis. Only 25 percent will be able to get rid of the virus on their own in the first 6 months.

Blood tests such as those for liver enzymes and viral load (amount of virus) do not always match the severity of the disease. For example, it is possible to have a low viral load or normal liver enzymes in a person with cirrhosis. Imaging studies such as CT scan or ultrasound can give the doctor some idea about the amount of liver damage. Liver biopsy (taking a small piece of the liver using a needle) is the gold standard to assess the amount of damage in the liver. The doctor may recommend biopsy for the person in your care.

Treatments are available for hepatitis C. You should talk to the doctor in detail about treatment to see if the person in your care is a good candidate for treatment. There is approximately a 30–50 percent chance that the person in your care can be cured of hepatitis C depending on the subtype of hepatitis C virus he has. Treatment may include weekly injections of interferon and taking pills called ribavirin daily.

Tip

The treatment has many side effects, but an experienced doctor can manage the side effects and help the patient with hepatitis C through treatment. Discuss possible side effects with the doctor.

The person who has hepatitis C should:

1. **Avoid alcohol consumption.** When a person with hepatitis C drinks alcohol it is like adding fuel to a fire. The person with hepatitis C can significantly reduce the chance of developing cirrhosis by staying away from alcohol. Encourage the person to join AA if he or she has a drinking problem.

2. **Avoid raw shellfish such as oysters, mussels, and clams.** Raw shellfish may contain certain bacteria that can cause liver infection. Sushi is OK for the person with hepatitis C.

3. **Never share toothbrushes or razors with others.**

It is important to make sure the doctor knows that the patient has hepatitis C prior to beginning any medication. Remember to always bring a complete list of medications to the doctor's visits and check with your liver specialist prior to starting any new medication or supplement.

> **NOTE** The virus can live outside the body for 1–2 days. It is important that you separate any items that can potentially come in contact with the infected person in your care and other people.

If the caregiver is the spouse or partner of the person who has HCV, it is important to discuss the use of a protective barrier such as a condom and HCV will not hinder your sexual relationship (see *Special Challenges,* page 161). Casual contact such as hugging and kissing is safe. There is no need for the person in your care to stay away from family and friends. It is also fine to share food from the same plate.

> **NOTE** You and the person in your care should get hepatitis A and B vaccines if not immune. There is no vaccine for hepatitis C.

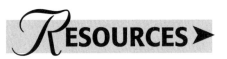

Centers for Disease Control – Hepatitis
www.cdc.gov/ncidod/diseases/hepatitis
Contains basic CDC information regarding hepatitis.

See page 12 for list of organizations for hepatitis information.

Cirrhosis and Its Complications

Cirrhosis and Its Complications

Cirrhosis

Cirrhosis is a word used to describe a liver that has a lot of scar tissue that replaces normal, healthy tissue. In a person with cirrhosis, the scar tissue in the liver prevents it from working like it should. Cirrhosis has multiple causes, but basically it's caused by chronic stress to the liver cells, leading to scar formation. Not all people with cirrhosis will require a liver transplant, but once a person develops symptoms of liver failure, the only option is a liver transplant. Cirrhosis is the twelfth leading cause of death by disease, killing about 26,000 people each year. In the United States, chronic alcoholism and hepatitis C are the most common causes of cirrhosis.

To understand the complications of cirrhosis, we have to first understand how the liver works. The liver removes poisons from the blood, makes substances that help with the immune system, and helps control sugar levels. It also makes proteins that regulate blood clotting and produces bile to help absorb fats and fat-soluble vitamins. The development of scar tissue in the liver is a process that takes place over years, and a lot of people with cirrhosis have no symptoms in the early stages of the disease. However, when the scar tissue impairs the function of healthy liver cells, liver function starts to fail, and the first signs of liver cirrhosis may begin to appear.

Some of the signs to watch for are—

- fatigue, weakness

- loss of appetite, weight loss

- nausea, vomiting

- abdominal pain; usually on upper right hand side of abdomen

- jaundice: yellowing of skin and eyes

- itching

- spider-like blood vessels (spider angiomas) that develop on the skin

It is important to understand that people with cirrhosis can experience a very wide range of possible symptoms. The person in your care can have a simple complaint like fatigue to severe confusion and life-threatening bleeding episodes.

 People with cirrhosis can have a wide range of disability— from being completely self-reliant and able to function to requiring assistance with the activities of daily living.

Complications

As cirrhosis progresses, more severe complications may develop. The caregiver should be aware of these conditions.

Ascites

Ascites (an accumulation of fluid in the peritoneal cavity [sac in the abdomen]) and edema (water accumulation in the stomach and legs) cause swelling in the abdomen and legs. The doctor may give the person in your care diuretic medication (water pill) to increase urination and reduce water retention.

 Salty foods lead to water retention. Avoid salt by being especially careful of choices when eating out and staying away from frozen, canned, and packaged foods.

Encephalopathy

Encephalopathy (confusion) is caused by a buildup of toxins in the blood that affect the brain, which leads to unresponsiveness, forgetfulness, trouble concentrating, or changes in sleep habits. This confusion usually comes on quickly, unlike dementia. The doctor will give the person in your care medicines to help with this if needed.

Tip

Lactulose is a medication often prescribed for confusion. Lactulose is also a laxative. The caregiver should measure this medication carefully so the person in care has 2–3 soft pudding like bowel movements on a daily basis.

Esophageal Varices

Esophageal varices (swollen or knotted blood vessels in the esophagus) occur because blood flow through the liver slows down due to scar tissue. This causes blood to back up into the blood vessels in the stomach and esophagus. Think of the vessels as a clogged drain; when a drain is clogged, water backs up. These blood vessels may become enlarged because they are not meant to carry this much blood. The enlarged blood vessels, called varices, have thin walls and carry high pressure, and thus are more likely to burst. If they do burst, the result is a serious bleeding problem in the upper stomach or esophagus that requires immediate medical attention.

Because this problem with blood backing up does not have any symptoms, it is important to check for these varices by doing EGD (esophagogastroduodenoscopy), which is a test that involves passing a scope (a tube with a light and a camera on one end) through the mouth into the esophagus to look for bulging veins. If found, the doctor can put rubber bands around the bulging vein to reduce the chance of bleeding. This procedure should be done every year if the person in your care has cirrhosis. However, in some cases it may be needed more often. There are also medicines that can be taken to decrease the pressure in these veins.

> **NOTE** Close monitoring of stool color should be done daily. Dark black stool can be a sign of internal bleeding, while pale colored stools may indicate jaundice (yellow color of skin).

Hepatocellular Carcinoma

Hepatocellular carcinoma is the medical term for cancer of the liver. This cancer is most often seen in patients with cirrhosis. The best treatment is a liver transplant, if possible. Patients will need to be referred to a liver transplant center for treatment and placement on a transplant list (see **Liver Transplant,** p. 27).

Cancer cannot be prevented in most cases. There are no symptoms in the early stages of cancer, so it is important to actively look for cancer by doing a blood test (AFP) and imaging studies (ultrasound, CT scan, or MRI) of the abdomen every six months. If found early, liver transplant is a very effective treatment for liver cancer. If found late, however, liver transplant may not be possible because getting on the transplant list is based on tumor size, the number of tumors, and evidence of the spread of cancer to other body parts.

There are helpful nutritional guidelines for patients with cirrhosis to help lessen and avoid these complications. These will be discussed in detail in **Diet, Nutrition, and Exercise,** p. 175.

Cirrhosis is an irreversible process, but often treatment can delay the worsening of liver disease and reduce complications. Treatment depends on the *cause* of cirrhosis, and targets specific complications that the person in your care is experiencing. When complications cannot be controlled or when the liver becomes so damaged from scarring that it completely stops functioning, a liver transplant is necessary. It is important that the person in your care see a hepatologist (liver specialist) or gastroenterologist (stomach and intestine specialist) for treatment recommendations early on to prevent cirrhosis.

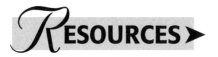
RESOURCES ➤

American Association for the Study of Liver Disease
www.aasld.org

American Liver Foundation
75 Maiden Lane
Suite 603
New York, NY 10038
(212) 668-1000 Fax: (212) 483-8179
www.liverfoundation.org

Liver Transplant

Liver Transplant

Liver transplant is the only treatment for people with liver failure. In some cases a liver transplant is also the best treatment for those with liver cancer. Therefore, when caring for a person with liver disease it is important to have some basic understanding of liver transplant. Transplantation is a complicated surgery during which the person's own diseased liver is removed and a new liver is placed into the body. This new liver can be from a deceased donor or from a live person who is willing to give half of his liver. The liver will grow back to normal size in both the donor and recipient (person getting the transplant) in one to two months.

> **NOTE** The liver is the only internal organ in the body with regenerating ability. Wow!

There are approximately 18,000 people currently waiting for a liver, but only 6,000 people get transplanted every year. The need for liver transplant is expected to increase in the next few years. As a result, the wait for liver transplant may become longer. The person in your care may become very sick before getting a liver. *While waiting for a liver, it is important to keep the person as healthy as possible.* Therefore, it is important for the caregiver to be aware of the complications of cirrhosis and help the person with liver disease manage the complications effectively (see *Cirrhosis and Its Complications,* p. 21); this will increase the ill person's quality of life. Caregivers have an important role in helping the person in care prevent complications by being actively involved in health care management.

When a person is found to have cirrhosis or complications of cirrhosis, it is recommended that he go through the liver transplant evaluation. The person with liver disease should have his health care managed by a hepatologist.

Choosing a Transplant Center

How do you choose a transplant center?

1. Often it is the insurance company that decides where the person in your care will go.

2. The person's gastroenterologist or primary care physician will also make a recommendation.

3. UNOS (United Network for Organ Sharing) will give information. Check with UNOS to see which center has had the best outcome.

The Evaluation

The evaluation process is long and detail oriented. This includes testing the liver as well as testing other important organs such as the heart, lungs, and kidneys. If the person with liver disease is found to be medically and psychologically fit for surgery, he becomes an eligible candidate and gets on the transplant waiting list. The caregiver has an important role in this process because most centers make sure the ill person has a caregiver who is willing to take care of the patient after surgery. The criteria for transplant are slightly different from center to center.

MELD Score

Unlike other types of organ transplant, liver transplant does not follow the philosophy of "first come, first served."

Rather, the new organ goes to the sickest person. This is decided based on a person's MELD (the Model for End-Stage Liver Disease) score, which is calculated by a blood test. The results of the test range from 6–40, 40 being the score of the sickest person. This system is controlled by UNOS, a branch of the government. The United States is divided into different regions. When an organ becomes available, it goes to the person with the highest MELD score in that region. The number of people waiting for liver transplant varies from region to region. Therefore, some areas have a shorter wait than others.

 Blood type also plays a role. Because blood type O is the most common blood group, there is a high demand for livers for people with this blood type. For this reason, there are more people with blood type O waiting for liver transplant compared to any other blood type.

Some people can get listed in more than one region to increase the chance of getting a transplant. Get more information by visiting the UNOS website (📖 see **Resources** p. 31).

Tip

Talk with the doctor during your visit to see if multiple listing is recommended for the person in your care. The caregiver plays an important role in learning more about transplants because most people needing liver transplants are too sick to look into this on their own.

After liver transplant, care receivers will be on multiple medications immediately. Some medicines are taken for life to prevent the body from rejecting the new liver. Rejection is a life-threatening event that happens when the patient's immune system sees the new liver as a foreign object and attacks it. These anti-rejection medicines keep the immune system less active and prevent rejection. It is important that the caregiver is actively involved in making sure that the transplant recipient takes the medicine correctly.

NOTE Do not forget to review the list of medicines with the liver patient's health care provider during each visit and clarify any questions or concerns you may have about them. The medicines have multiple side effects. Discuss all symptoms so the doctor can decide if any of the medicines need to be changed to reduce the risk of long-term effects or damage.

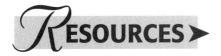

RESOURCES ➤

United Network for Organ Sharing (UNOS)
P. O. Box 2484
Richmond, VA 23218
(804) 782-4800 Fax: (804) 782-4817
Patient info: (888) 894-6361
www.unos.org
The UNOS oversees the database of transplant information and operates the organ sharing system, matching donors and recipients.

Using the Health Care Team Effectively

Using the Health Care Team Effectively

*W*hen you care for someone in the home, you must also manage that person's health care. This means choosing a good medical team, keeping costs down, arranging for medical appointments, and getting the best, least expensive medicines. It also means knowing what the insurance rules are and, most important, being an advocate (a supporter) for the person in your care.

Doctors and nurses can focus on physical diagnosis and may ignore the emotional aspects of care. Sometimes they have little time to consider the spiritual aspects of healing. Although you should consult with professionals about the levels of therapy and support needed for the person in your care, you do not have to accept what they suggest or order. Keep asking questions until you completely understand the diagnosis (what is wrong), treatment, and prognosis (likely outcome).

Choosing a Doctor

Call your local medical society for the names of doctors who specialize in the field in which you seek care. Think about using doctors who are allied with transplant centers. They tend to have the most up-to-date information, especially about complicated illnesses.

- Always make sure the doctor is board certified in his or her specialty.

- If the person in your care is enrolled in an HMO, ask if the particular transplant center will accept the HMO insurance.

- You can contact more than one doctor or transplant center (for a second opinion). If you are enrolled in

Medicare Supplementary Medical Insurance (Part B), Medicare will pay for a second opinion in the same way it pays for other services. After Part B of the deductible has been met, Medicare pays 80 percent of the Medicare-approved amount for a second opinion and will provide the same coverage for a third opinion.

Nurse Practitioners/Physician Assistants

Seek out a medical practice that incorporates the services of a nurse practitioner or physician assistant. These mid-level practitioners provide health screening, perform physical examinations, order laboratory tests, and prescribe specific medications authorized by the physician. Nurse practitioners/physician assistants also educate patients about staying healthy. Often they are the best-equipped health professionals to educate patients and caregivers about the common problems of chronic illness. Mid-level health care providers usually spend more time with patients and care-givers than the supervising medical specialists in a busy practice.

How to Share in Medical Decisions

In the end, medical decision-making is in the hands of the person receiving care, the doctor, and the caregiver. Learn to take an active role and become an advocate for yourself and for the person in your care. It has been said that a patient is the senior partner in the patient–doctor relationship.

Long-Range Considerations

- Find out how the person in your care feels about treatments that prolong life. Respect these views.

- Help the person receiving care to set up an advance directive and power of attorney for health care.

• Share decisions with the doctor and the care receiver and take responsibility for the treatment and its outcomes.

The Doctor–Patient–Caregiver Relationship

• Be aware that doctors must see more patients per day than they once did.

• Specialists are often the only ones with the training needed to treat a serious or chronic condition, so the doctor may refer the care receiver to a specialist or transplant center.

• If the relationship with the doctor becomes unfriendly, find a new doctor.

• Respect the doctor's time (you may need to have more than one visit to cover all issues).

• If Medicare is the payer, ask if the doctor accepts Medicare assignment. If not, the difference may have to be paid out of pocket.

Preparing for a Visit to the Doctor

• Be prepared to briefly explain the care receiver's and the family's medical history.

• Bring a list of medications currently taken by the person in your care.

• Take a list of questions in order of importance.

• Prepare a list of any symptoms the person you care for is experiencing.

- Be prepared to ask for written information on the medical situation so you can better understand what the doctor is saying, or bring a small tape recorder.

- You can call the hospital's library or health resource center for help in looking up any questions the doctor does not answer.

 Be sure shots for tetanus, flu, and pneumonia are up-to-date. For those on Medicare, flu and pneumonia shots are covered.

At the Doctor's Office

- Tell the doctor what you hope and expect from the visit and any recommended treatment.

- If the doctor tells you to do something you know you can't do, such as give medication in the middle of the night, ask if there is another treatment and explain why.

- Insist on talking about the level of care that you believe is appropriate and that agrees with the care receiver's wishes.

- Ask about other options for tests, medications, and surgery.

- Ask why tests or treatments are needed and what the risks are.

- Consider all options, including the pros and cons of "watchful waiting."

- Trust your common sense and, if you have doubts, get a second opinion.

Checklist Changes to Report to the Doctor

Contact the doctor right away if the following changes occur. Fever may be caused by an infection and should always be reported:

Diet

✓ extreme thirst

✓ lack of thirst

✓ weight loss for no reason

✓ loss of appetite

✓ pain before or after eating

✓ difficulty chewing or swallowing

Behavior

✓ unusual tiredness or sleepiness

✓ unusual actions (arguing, fighting, anger, or withdrawal)

✓ seeing or hearing things that aren't there (hallucinations)

✓ anxiety

✓ increased confusion

✓ depression

✓ inappropriate or unusual emotions

Bowel/Bladder

✓ bowel movements of an odd color, texture, or amount

✓ feeling faint during bowel movements

✓ pain when going to the bathroom (unusual color, amount, or odor)

✓ having to go to the bathroom frequently

✓ frequent bladder infections

✓ blood in the urine

✓ pain in the kidney area

✓ blood in the stool

✓ black stool

Skin

✓ changes in the color of lips, nails, fingers, and toes

✓ odd skin (color, temperature, texture, bruises)

✓ unusual appearance of surgery incisions

✓ sudden skin rashes (bumps, itching)

✓ pressure sores (bedsores)

Bones, Muscles, and Joints

✓ swelling in the legs

Chest

✓ chest pain

✓ rapid pulse

✓ painful breathing (wheezing, shortness of breath)

✓ unusual cough

✓ unusual saliva or mucus (report color and consistency)

✓ for male patients, painful breasts as well as swelling of the breasts

Abdomen

✓ stomach pain

✓ vomiting

✓ increased abdominal girth

Head

✓ dizziness

✓ headaches

✓ ear pain, discharge, or change in hearing

✓ mouth sores

✓ nose pain (bleeding, bad odor to mucus)

KEEP ASKING QUESTIONS UNTIL YOU ARE SATISFIED. Doctors and other health care professionals have medical know-how, but only you can explain symptoms. Report exactly, in as few words as possible, any unusual symptoms, changes in condition, and complaints the person has.

If the Person in Your Care Is Near Death

Because few doctors are trained to talk about death and the dying process with their patients, be prepared to begin the conversation.

- If the person in your care wants to die at home, say this clearly to the doctor.

- Be sure that any directives for health care for the person are available and prominently displayed.

Questions to Ask Before Agreeing to Tests, Medications, and Surgery

Before you begin discussing medical treatment with the doctor, explain that the person in your care does not want any unnecessary tests or treatments. Then ask these questions:

- Why is this test needed?

- How long will it take? How soon will the results be in?

- Is the test accurate?

- Is it painful?

- Are there risks with the treatment? Do the benefits outweigh the risks?

- How long will side effects occur and how long will they last?

- Will the doctor review the test report and explain it in detail?

- May a copy of the report be taken home? (If you have questions, ask to talk to the specialist who made the report.)

- If a test is positive, what course of action should be taken?

- Is the condition going to worsen slowly or rapidly?

- What could happen if the person did not have the test?

- How much does the test cost and is there a less costly one that will give the same information?

Liver Disease and Medications

Questions to Ask the Doctor About Medications

Medications can be costly, confusing to use, and have unwanted side effects. Be sure to ask questions when medicines are prescribed and prescriptions are filled.

- Give the doctor a list of all medications and dosages that the person in your care is now taking, including eye drops, vitamins, herbal remedies, and over-the-counter medicines.

- Tell the doctor of any allergies or if there are certain foods the person cannot eat (food allergies). Find out about any allergies including common ones and dangerous ones.

- How long should a particular medicine be taken? Is it long term or short term?

- Try to find the drug at the lowest cost. Ask if a generic (nonbrand name) drug or another brand in the same drug class is available at a lower cost.

- Be sure that the generic drug will not have a poor effect on the person's condition.

- To keep costs down, ask if a higher dose can be safely prescribed and the pill cut in half.

Diuretics (water pills)

Furosemide (Lasix®) and spironolactone (Aldactone®) are the most commonly used water pills. They help reduce swelling in the legs and abdomen by ridding the body of excess water. They are more efficient when used together. They also offset the potassium imbalance each medication creates. If one medicine is reduced or increased, it is important to ask the doctor about the person in your care's potassium balance. It is dangerous if her potassium level gets too low. Water pills are hard on the kidneys. When on these medicines it is important that the person is monitored closely by the doctor and has blood tests.

Increased urination is a common effect of these medicines. The person will likely have to urinate during the night, which causes sleep disturbance. Ask the doctor if the person in your care can take the pills in the morning (once a day) or in the afternoon, around 3.00 P.M., if the pills need to be taken twice a day. Avoid having her take them later at night so she might not have to wake up to urinate.

If the swelling does not go away, make sure to notify the doctor so any necessary changes can be made to the prescription.

Breast enlargement or tenderness is also a side effect of spironolactone. This can be a problem for male patients. Discuss this with the doctor. Another medicine can be prescribed safely to replace spironolactone. It is called amiloride. Do not stop these medicines because of the side effects unless directed by the doctor.

Beta blocker

Propanolol (Inderal®) or nadolol is used to decrease the internal pressure and reduce varicose veins in the esophagus and stomach. This is important to prevent the veins bursting and bleeding. Dizziness is a common side effect of this medicine. Report side effects to the doctor so he or she can make necessary changes or adjust the dose.

Lactulose

This is a sweet syrup used to decrease toxic buildup in the brain that can lead to confusion (hepatic encephalopathy). One of the major side effects of this medicine is diarrhea. Do not stop the medicine if the person in care gets diarrhea. Adjust the dose (increase or decrease the dose) so he has three to four soft bowel movements per day. Tell the doctor if confusion does not go away with this medicine. The doctor may add other medicine to help.

 These medicines are used to control the complications of cirrhosis. They are not medicines used to treat the *underlying liver* disease. Some types of liver disease are treatable and some are not. Talk to the doctor about these medications.

 BUYING MEDICATIONS
Buying medications through mail order is often the cheapest way to buy. Ask if the insurance company has a mail-order program (📖 see **Resources,** p. 52).

Questions to Ask the Pharmacist

Some prescription drugs are not covered by health insurance, so shop around for the drug store with the lowest prices, and then stay with it. The pharmacist will come to know the care receiver's condition and can advise you about problems that might come up. Managed care plans are permitted to change doctor's orders by giving you a similar version of a drug that is cheaper. Do not try cutting drug costs without talking to the doctor about it first.

- Find out the highest allowable price that can be charged for a particular drug.

- Ask if the doctor can be called to approve the switch to another drug.

- Find out what generic drug can be used instead of the name-brand drug.

- Ask if using more than one drug can cause unsafe drug interactions.

- Find out the risks of not taking the medicine.

- Find out the risks of not finishing the prescription.

- If you are caring for someone who will be taking several medications on her own, find a drug store that has easy-to-open pill bottles.

- Ask if the medicine can be put in a large easy-to-open container with a label in large print.

- Find a pharmacy that is open 24/7.

- Ask if the medicine must be taken with a meal, with water or milk, etc.

- When the person in care needs many expensive drugs, find out if you can get a discount or work out a payment plan.

 Tip

MEDICAL ALERT
People with liver disease may want to wear a medical alert bracelet, or carry a card that lists the medications he or she is currently taking.

Questions to Ask About Surgery

Sometimes it is necessary for people with cirrhosis to undergo a surgical procedure. Any surgery in these people has increased risks. Abdominal surgery is even riskier and therefore should be done only by a liver transplant surgeon. Surgery is a serious step. Ask as many questions as you need before deciding to go ahead.

- Why does the person need the surgery?

- Will the surgery stop the problem or merely slow it down?

- What are the other choices?

- Can it be done on an outpatient basis?

- What will happen if surgery is not done?

- Where will the surgery be done? When?

- Will the surgeon you spoke to do the surgery or will it be assigned to another doctor? (When going into surgery, put the surgeon's name on the release form to ensure that the named surgeon is the one who does the operation.)

- How many surgeries of this type has the doctor performed? (Generally, the more times the surgeon has performed an operation, the higher the success rate will be.)

- What is the doctor's success rate with this type of surgery?

- What are the anesthesiologist's qualifications?

- What can go wrong?

- How much will the surgery cost, and is it covered by insurance?

>
>
> **MEDICAL RECORDS**
>
> If going for a second opinion: to save costs, have all medical records and tests sent to the second doctor. Also, if possible, bring the important ones with you. Even the experts can disagree about the best treatment. The final decision is yours.

Alternative Treatments

A healthy lifestyle is encouraged by most medical providers. Use caution if you decide to try a different kind of treatment (known as complementary or alternative treatment). Look before you leap and follow these commonsense guidelines:

- Be on guard against anyone who says to stop seeing a conventional (regular) doctor or to stop taking prescribed medicine.

- Look into the background of any treatment provider.

- Discuss the alternative or complementary therapy with your doctor.

- Figure out the costs of the treatments.

- Do not abandon conventional therapy.

- Keep a written account of the experience.

Mental Health Treatment

Strong emotions are a normal part of long-term illness and some medications used to treat chronic hepatitis can worsen depression. Counseling and support groups are a very helpful way of dealing with these feelings.

- For one who is depressed and needs therapy, ask the primary care doctor to give you the name of a therapist.

- Be aware that many people are embarrassed about mental health problems and may not want to seek care.

- For help determining a person's ability to make legal decisions, arrange for a psychiatrist's assessment.

How to Watch Out for Someone's Best Interests in the Hospital

A person in the hospital is at greater risk than others, so be ready to keep tabs on treatments, ask questions, and act as an advocate.

- If the Patients' Bill of Rights is not posted in a place where it can be seen, ask for a copy.

- Agree only to treatments that have been thoroughly explained.

- If something is not being done and you think it should be, ask why.

- Be friendly and show respect to hospital staff. They will probably respond better to you and to the person in your care. Bad feelings between family members and staff may cause the staff to avoid the person.

- Assist with the person's grooming and care.

- Speak up if you notice doctors or nurses examining anyone without first washing their hands.

- Check all bills and ask questions about anything that isn't clear to you.

NOTE According to federal law, a hospital must release patients in a *safe manner* or else must keep them in the hospital. Letting a patient leave the hospital is not wise if the person has constant fever, infection or pain that cannot be controlled, confusion, disorientation (no sense of time or place), or is unable to take food and liquids by mouth. However, in some cases, it may be better for the person to be released because the noise and risk of catching other diseases may make it more difficult to recover. If you plan to appeal a discharge, understand the rules of Medicare, Medicaid, the HMO, or insurance plan.

When You Doubt the Time Is Right for Discharge

- State your doubts in a simple letter to the hospital's director or the health plan's medical director. (Rules vary from state to state.)

- Meet with the hospital's discharge planner.

- Ask if the hospital is following the usual policy for the condition.

- Explain any special reasons that make you think it is unwise to discharge the person.

- Ask if the hospital rules can be changed to cover this special case.

- Remember that anyone has the right to appeal a discharge.

- Get your doctor's help in the appeal, but understand that he or she may have different reasons for wanting to discharge the person.

Checklist Coming Home from the Hospital

✓ Assess the person's condition and needs.

✓ Understand the diagnosis (what is wrong) and prognosis (what will happen).

✓ Become part of the health care team (doctor, nurse, therapists) so you can learn how to provide care.

✓ Get complete written instructions from the doctor. If there is anything you don't understand, ASK QUESTIONS.

✓ Arrange follow-up care from the doctor.

✓ Develop a plan of care with the doctor. (📖 See **Setting Up a Plan of Care,** p. 107.)

✓ Meet with the hospital's social worker or discharge planner to determine home care benefits.

✓ Understand in-home assistance options.

✓ Arrange for in-home help.

✓ Arrange physical, occupational, and speech therapy as needed.

✓ Find out if medicine is provided by the hospital to take home. If not, you will have to have prescriptions filled before you take the person home.

✓ Prepare the home. (📖 See **Preparing the Home,** p. 87.)

✓ Buy needed supplies; rent, borrow, or buy equipment such as wheelchairs, crutches, and walkers.

✓ Take home all personal items.

✓ Check with the hospital cashier for discharge payment requirements.

✓ Arrange transportation (an ambulance or van if your car will not do).

NOTE Do not hesitate to call the hospital staff member (ombudsman) who is responsible for patients' rights.

Case Management

Case management is an important resource for families living with chronic illness. It is easy to become stressed out with the demands of the disease and with the red tape of the health care and social services network. Case managers need to have a basic understanding of the special needs of persons with chronic illness.

Case management skills are very helpful to families when there is a change in the person's physical state or in awareness and understanding. Should this happen, a case manager can take another look at the person's needs and at community supports. This may be necessary in the following instances:

- when the person loses the ability to process information and help is needed to identify issues and provide follow-up with a course of action

- when there is a change in the caregiver situation or support network that can easily become a crisis for the family as a whole

- when there are fewer financial resources and the family is no longer able to pay for the resources they need

- when safety issues arise that can put the ill person at greater risk

These issues and others require that case management continue as a long-term resource, so that the case manager can step in when needed to provide more support.

To learn more about case management or find a case manager in your area, contact:

- your local Visiting Nurse Association

- hospital discharge planners

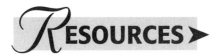

For free or low-cost resources, contact local consumer health resource and information centers (check the local hospital system or phone book) and local health agencies or associations (American Heart Association, American Diabetes Association, National Multiple Sclerosis Society, and others).

Doctor's Guide to the Internet—Patient Edition
www.pslgroup.com/PTGUIDE.HTM
Provides information for specific diseases and gives pointers to other Internet sites of medical information.

Go Ask Alice!
www.goaskalice.columbia.edu/about.html
Provides helpful information and lets you post health-related questions.

The Health Resource, Inc.
933 Faulkner Street
Conway, AR 72034
(800) 949-0090; (501) 329-5272; Fax (501) 329-9489
www.thehealthresource.com
Provides clients with personalized detailed reports on their specific medical conditions. These reports contain conventional and alternative treatments and information on current research, nutrition, self-help measures, specialists, and resource organizations. Reports on any non-cancer condition are $295, or $395 for complex issues, and contain 50 to 100 pages. Reports on any cancer condition are $395 and contain 150 to 200 pages. Shipping is additional.

University of Washington
www.uwmedicine.org
A great storehouse of general health information on all topics.

Medications

Together Rx Access® Card
A joint program by drug companies offering a free Prescription Savings Card for individuals and families who meet all four of the following requirements:

❏ *Not eligible for Medicare*

❏ *Have no public or private prescription drug coverage*

❏ *Household income equal to or less than:*

—$30,000 for a single person
—$40,000 for a family of two
—$50,000 for a family of three
—$60,000 for a family of four
—$70,000 for a family of five

❏ *Legal resident of the U.S. or Puerto Rico*

Call 1-800-250-2839 to start saving on your prescriptions. For the most current list of medicines and products, visit www.TogetherRxAccess.com

Publication

A Family Caregiver's Guide to Hospital Discharge Planning, a publication of the National Alliance for Caregiving and the United Hospital Fund of New York.
Available at www.caregiving.org

If you don't have access to the Internet, ask your local library to help you locate a Web site.

Paying for Care

❦

Paying for Care

$\mathcal{Y}$ ou can look to many sources for help in paying for care. Some are public, while others are private or volunteer. The most common ways to pay for home care are as follows:

- *personal and family resources*

- *private insurance*

- *Medicare, Medicaid, Department of Veterans Affairs, and Title programs*

- *community-based services*

Assessment of Financial Resources

First, complete a personal financial resources assessment by doing the following steps:

- Look at current assets, where your income comes from, and insurance entitlements.

- Prepare a budget and figure out what your future income might be from all sources.

- Confirm the qualifications, retirement benefits, and Social Security status of the person in your care.

- Figure as closely as possible the expenses of professional care and equipment. Include any medical procedures likely to be needed.

- Check on the person's personal tax status and find out what care items and expenses are deductible.

- Find out if the person's health insurance or employer's workers' compensation policy has home health care benefits.

- Figure out how much money the person will need.

 Think about making the person in your care a "dependent" and thus be able to transfer medical expenses to a taxpayer who can make use of medical deductions.

Public Pay Programs

Medicare

Medicare is a federal health insurance program. It provides health care benefits to all Americans 65 and older and to those who have been determined to be "disabled" according to the Social Security Administration. After an individual has received Social Security Disability benefits for two years, he becomes eligible for Medicare benefits regardless of age. There are constant changes in Medicare policies, requirements, and forms. Therefore, it is always best to get the most current information on benefits by calling the Medicare Hotline (see p. 70) or your hospital's social worker.

Things That Affect Medicare Eligibility

Whether the Person Is Homebound—Medicare will pay for certain home health care services only if the person is confined to the home and requires part-time skilled (nursing) services or therapy. Medicare does not cover ongoing custodial (maintenance) care. "Confined to home" does not mean bedridden. It means that a person cannot leave home except for medical care and requires help to get there. (Brief absences from the home do not affect eligibility.)

In order for treatments, services, and supplies to be paid, they must be ordered by a doctor. They must also be provided by a home health agency certified by Medicare and the state health department.

Whether Care Is Intermittent (periodic)—In order to be covered, skilled services are required. Medicare is not designed to meet chronic ongoing needs that are considered "custodial" rather than "skilled."

Medicare Generally Pays for the Following:

- almost all costs of skilled care, such as doctors, nurses, and specialists

- various types of therapy—occupational, physical, speech-language

- home health services

- medical supplies and equipment

- personal care by home health aides (such as bathing, dressing, fixing meals, even light housekeeping and counseling) after discharge from a hospital or nursing home

Medicare Part D–Prescription Drug Plan

Beginning January 1, 2006, Medicare covers prescription drugs. There are two basic ways to sign up for this coverage. If you have traditional Medicare (Part A for hospital services and Part B for doctor and outpatient health-care providers), you may sign up for a stand-alone Medicare Part D prescription drug plan. You can also choose a managed care plan under Medicare Advantage. These plans restrict you to only the doctors on the managed-care provider's list. They also have a prescription drug plan. All plans are from private companies that have been approved by Medicare (📖 see *Resources* p. 70).

Help is available to pay for copayments and premiums for those whose incomes are low enough to be eligible. A person must apply to the Social Security Administration for financial assistance.

> **NOTE** Phrases like "intermittent care," "skilled care," and "homebound" are not precisely defined. They are different from region to region, and the type and availability of coverage by Medicare may be different as well.

Services NOT covered by Medicare

Full-time nursing care at home, drugs, meals delivered to the home, homemaker chore services not related to care, and personal care services are usually not covered by Medicare.

> **NOTE** A caregiver who has power of attorney for a person on Medicare (the beneficiary) must send written permission to the person's Medicare Part B carrier. Send a letter with the person's name, number, signature, and a statement that the caregiver can act on behalf of the beneficiary. The form must list start and end dates.
>
> If there is a dispute about a repayment from Medicare, a review may be requested by filing a claim with the Medicare carrier.

Medicare Part B Insurance

Medicare Part B insurance costs between $96 and $238 per month (2008) and is based on yearly income. It offers extra benefits to basic Medicare coverage. It pays for tests, doctor's office visits, lab services, and home health care. A $135 deductible applies (2008). Medicare Parts A and B also cover some costs of organ transplantation.

Medicare Supplemental Insurance (Medigap)

To pay for benefits not covered by Medicare, this private health insurance option is available. It pays for noncovered services only—for example, hospital deductibles, doctor copayments, and eyeglasses—but does not cover long-term care services. Coverage depends on the plan you buy.

For anyone who has Medicare HMO coverage, Medigap insurance may not be necessary because those individuals only make a small copayment but do not pay a deductible for doctor's visits.

 It is illegal for an insurance company or agent to sell you a second Medigap policy unless you put in writing that you intend to end the Medigap policy you have. The federal toll-free telephone number for filing complaints is (800) 633-4227.

Medicaid

Medicaid pays for the medical care of low-income persons or those whose assets have been used up while paying for their own care. Eligibility depends on monthly income limits and personal assets. Coverage includes nursing facilities, assisted living, foster care, and certain types of home care. Each state runs its own Medicaid program, and so eligibility and coverage can vary. Some states have set up Medicaid Waiver programs, which pay for home and community-based services that would otherwise only be paid if one were in a nursing home.

Common Aspects of Medicaid

- Recipients must be financially and medically in need.

- For recipients who are terminally ill, benefits go on for as long as they are ill. However, care must be provided by an agency with hospice certification and Medicaid certification.

- Payments are made directly to providers of services.

- Long-term-care costs are paid for those not covered by insurance and for patients whose finances have run out.

- Payments to foster care homes and retirement communities are not covered (except in some cases by Medicaid waiver).

- Home health care services, medical supplies, and equipment are covered.

- Eligibility is based on a person's income and assets.

- People with disabilities who are eligible for state public assistance are eligible for Medicaid.

- People with disabilities eligible for Supplemental Social Security (SSI) are eligible for Medicaid.

- In many states, there are laws (called spousal impoverishment laws) that protect a portion of the estate and assets for the healthy spouse. These come into play after other monies have been "spent down" for the care of the ill spouse.

To find out what the benefits are, contact the local Social Security office, city or county public assistance office, or the Area Agency on Aging.

Services NOT covered by Medicaid

As a rule, Medicare, Medicaid, and private insurance do not cover many in-home services because they are not medical services. However, some community services may be called on to fill the gap for free or on a subsidized (public funding) basis. The following services usually are not covered but might be available locally free of charge:

- adult day care

- case management

- household chore services

- neighborhood and local meal services, such as Meals on Wheels

- consumer protection

- emergency response systems (which provide contact by phone or electronic device to police and rescue services)

- emergency assistance for food, clothing, or shelter

- friendly visitors (volunteers who stop by to write letters or run errands)

- services and equipment for those who have disabilities

- homemaker services

- legal and financial services

- respite care

- senior centers

- support groups (which will send materials if you write to them)

- telephone reassurance (volunteers who make calls to or receive calls from those who are elderly or living alone)

The U.S. Congress and the Administration made major changes to Medicare and Medicaid, which will affect payment for long-term care. As these changes are put into effect, they are posted on the Web site of the Center for Medicare and Medicaid Services (CMS): www.cms.gov

Department of Veterans Affairs Benefits

Veterans generally qualify for health services in the home if a disability is service related. Even if a disability is not service related, other benefits may be available based on income qualifications. Some states have special programs only for veterans who live in that state. Some Veterans Hospitals have programs to deliver home health care services. Contact the nearest Veterans Affairs office or veterans group in your area.

Older Americans Act and Social Services Block Grant

Some agencies that provide support services get funding under this program. Services available may include the following:

- case management and assessment
- household chore services (minor household repairs, cleaning, yard work)
- companion services
- community meals
- home-delivered hot meals (Meals on Wheels) once or twice a day
- homemaker services
- transportation

Private Pay Long-Term-Care Insurance

Generally, private insurance programs do not cover long-term care. In many cases, home care reimbursement is severely restricted or prohibited. Policies must be examined closely. Before buying long-term care insurance, seek the best, most knowledgeable help available on the subject (for example, consult a hospital discharge planner or the Area Agency on Aging). Seek agents who represent reliable companies and have a reputation for honesty. The lack of uniformity in long-term care policies makes it hard to compare them.

- Policies vary greatly so don't assume one is like another you are familiar with.

- It's important to read the fine print.

- Such policies should not be considered an option for anyone over 79.

- Coverage is often limited to Medicare-certified nursing homes.

- Sometimes benefits are provided for hospice care for the terminally ill.

- Benefits are usually $50–$200 per day.

- A typical policy for a healthy 65-year-old costs about $3,000 per year.

- Long-term-care insurance should be purchased before age 60, when premiums are relatively low.

- Some policies offer direct cash for home care instead of reimbursement (so payment can be used for a family caregiver).

- It is important to buy what you can comfortably afford.

Checklist **Long–Term–Care Insurance Policies**

✓ Look for an insurer that is top rated by Moody's Investors Service, A.M. Best Company, or Standard & Poor's Corporation.

✓ Find out how long the company has been in business and check the Better Business Bureau or the state's Insurance Division for complaints.

✓ Take someone with you when you meet the agent.

✓ Never pay cash to an agent. The payment should be made by check written to the insurance company and be sure the agent gives you a signed and dated receipt when the policy is delivered.

✓ Find premiums that do not exceed 5–6% of the covered individual's income.

✓ Ask for an "Outline of Coverage" which the law requires the insurance company to provide even if you do not want to fill out an application for insurance. Use this outline to compare policies.

✓ Understand how and when you can contact the care manager.

✓ Look for a policy that pays for care at home, in any adult foster care home, assisted living facility, and nursing home (not just one that is Medicare certified).

✓ Avoid policies that cover only skilled care. Look for policies that allow respite care and adult day care.

✓ Find out when the insurance pays for home custodial care or hospice care.

✓ Find out if previous hospitalization, a nursing home stay, or other restrictive eligibility criteria are required.

✓ Be sure that benefits will increase with inflation.

✓ Make sure that benefits last at least three years if you don't buy lifetime benefits.

✓ Find out if some coverage is provided if the policy lapses and what conditions must be met before benefits can be started.

✓ Make sure the policy is guaranteed renewable regardless of age.

✓ Get several proposals before making a decision.

Long-term-care insurance has two parts:

- In-home care benefits, which usually pay $100 per day for personal and domestic chores provided by a licensed home health agency.

- Nursing home benefits of approximately $200 a day.

To activate a policy, the policy holder must get confirmation from a doctor that he or she has lost the ability to do two or more of the following: bathing, eating, dressing, moving without falling, going to the toilet, and moving from a bed to a chair. The insurance company will send its representative to confirm the diagnosis. Homemaker benefits usually do not go into effect until 60 to 100 days after a hospital stay, and strict criteria must be met before in-home help is provided.

Consider Long-Term-Care Insurance If:

- Personal assets exceed $100,000 for a couple or $50,000 for a single person and need to be protected.

- The assets cannot be transferred.

- There is a family history of frail elderly.

- No one will be available to care for the person.

 Many states license individuals to offer analysis of insurance coverage for a fee. In some states if a person has a license to sell and a license to counsel, he or she can only perform one of those services for a specific client. Check your state department of insurance for information about insurance counselors.

Health Maintenance Organizations (HMOs)

Health Maintenance Organizations are prepaid health insurance plans that give complete medical coverage for a fixed premium. Knowing whether an HMO is right for the person in your care requires careful study.

Types of HMOs

There are three types of HMOs:

IPA (Individual Practice Associations) Plans—A patient chooses a doctor from a primary care physician list.

POS (Point of Service) Plans—For an extra fee a patient can visit a doctor outside of the network list.

Group Model HMOs—A patient must go to a clinic for treatment.

Remember, HMOs receive the same fees to treat a healthy person as a person with a chronic disease. For some patients with long-term or chronic illness, HMOs may not be a good choice. A patient who has a long-established relationship with a specialist who is not a member of the HMO's network list may not be able to continue to see that specialist.

 If a Medicare health plan is not meeting the needs of the person in your care, it is not difficult to switch to another plan or to a fee-for-service program.

How To Determine If an HMO Is Right for the Person in Your Care

- Ask if the doctor or specialist the person is now seeing is in the HMO network.

- Understand the person's medical needs—for special equipment, drugs, and help with activities. Determine if these needs are covered.

- Find out if the HMO is used to dealing with the illness the person has.

- Determine the specific services offered for this type of illness.

- Ask who decides what is medically necessary.

- Ask if there is a special Plan of Care for the illness.

- Ask if the person will get the *best* drugs for the condition or if generic substitutes will be offered.

- Ask how many people with this type of illness are under the plan in your area.

- Verify that the patient may see the specialists listed in the directory.

- Ask if the plan allows visits to specialists without a primary care doctor's referral.

- If a referral is required, find out how long it lasts and if a new referral is required for every visit.

- Ask what percentage of doctors on the list are board certified (have passed a special test given by the board of their specialty).

- Ask if the doctor has a financial incentive to do tests or to keep the patient from having tests or seeing a specialist.

- Ask if the plan covers visits to doctors outside the plan's referral list. (Out-of-network coverage may be limited to a certain dollar amount.)

- Ask how many doctors in the HMO specialize in geriatric care.

- If the person in your care must travel to a specific locale for extended stays, be sure the HMO allows visits to a different HMO there.

- Ask how the person will be charged if an emergency room visit is needed while traveling.

- Ask about the process for appealing a medical decision.

- Once you have decided on an HMO, get confirmation in writing regarding the items or services that are most important to the person in your care.

 To find out how many patient complaints were registered against an HMO, call your state insurance commissioner in the phone book under State Government.

How to Appeal an HMO's Decision Regarding a Medical Procedure, Prescription, or Specialist Referral

When a treatment is denied, the goal is to reverse the denial as quickly as possible. Remember that the HMO can prolong a case in court, so the goal is to resolve the case without litigation.

- Call the HMO and ask for a copy of its formal appeals process. (Federal law requires HMOs to have such a process.)

- Make detailed notes of all conversations with the HMO; include the date and the staff person's name.

- Determine exactly why the HMO refused to cover the treatment.

- Ask the HMO clerk for an explanation; if the matter is not resolved, ask for the HMO medical director's explanation of denial of treatment.

- If you still feel the situation is not resolved, start a written appeal process.

- Ask the doctor for a written explanation why treatment is medically necessary (also ask the specialists you have visited for a letter of support).

- Save all bills related to the problem.

- For consumer advice or support for the appeal, call the state insurance department, state health department, advocacy group for the disease, or local Area Agency on Aging.

> *Tip*
>
> The clerk at the other end of the line is a person too, and being courteous always gets a better response than being viewed as irrational or disrespectful.

Community-Based Services

Many services are provided free by local or community groups. The groups are sometimes repaid by state, local, and federal governments, but often volunteers provide meals and social and health care services.

These services can sometimes make it possible for a person to stay at home and maintain independence.

Typical Services

Community-based services include the following:

Adult Day Care Centers, which provide services ranging from health assessment to social programs that help people with dementia or those at risk for nursing home placement.

Nutrition Sites, which serve meals in settings such as senior centers, housing projects, faith-based centers, and schools and sometimes provide transportation.

Meals on Wheels, which brings healthful food to the home.

Senior Centers, which offer a place to socialize and eat. (Often a hot meal at noontime on weekdays is the only one served.)

Transportation is offered by hospitals, nursing homes, local governments, and religious, civic, or other groups. Out-of-pocket costs vary and fees are set on a sliding scale based on ability to pay.

Do These Services Meet Your Needs?

For whatever need you have, there is most likely a program in your area. Here are some things to think about:

- Is the person the right age and income level to be eligible for the program?

- Is it necessary for the person to belong to a certain organization to be eligible?

- Is there a limit to how many times the person can use the services of the organization?

Where to Check

- local agencies (Catholic Charities, United Way, Jewish Family and Child Services, Lutheran Family Services)

- local churches, parishes, or congregations

- the government blue book pages under public service listings

- city or county public assistance offices

- rural areas (call the health agency in the county seat)

- personal doctor

- family services department

- hospital discharge planner or social worker

- insurance company

- local Area Agency on Aging

- previous or current employer (may have benefits)

- public health department

- Social Security office

- state insurance commission

- state or local ombudsman

The Area Agency on Aging can help find services in the community. It will know whether chore services, home-delivered meals, friendly visitors, and telephone reassurance are free of charge or are provided on a sliding scale.

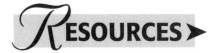 **RESOURCES ➤**

AARP
601 E. Street, NW
Washington, D.C. 20049
(800) 424-3410
www.aarp.org
Provides information on Medicare beneficiaries.

Centers for Medicare and Medicaid Services
7500 Security Boulevard
Baltimore, MD 21244-1850
(800) MEDICARE (633-4227) Medicare Hotline
www.cms.gov
www.medicare.gov

Federal agency that administers the Medicare and Medicaid programs, including hospice benefits.

National Association of Professional Geriatric Care Managers
1604 N. Country Club Road
Tucson, AZ 85716
(520) 881-8008
www.caremanager.org
Their Web site provides a free list of care managers in your state.

The National Council on the Aging
300 D Street SW, Suite 801
Washington, D.C. 20024
(202) 479-1200
www.ncoa.org
Provides a link to benefits (www.benefitscheckup.org) that helps seniors find state and federal benefits programs.

If you don't have access to the Internet, ask your local library to help you locate a Web site.

Financial Management and Tax Planning

Financial Management and Tax Planning

*T*here are many legal tools and tax tips that can help you and the person in your care now and in the future. Financial and life planning are necessary and should be started early. Long-term planning will help the caregiver feel more secure, no matter what the future brings. Life planning includes looking at income tax issues, protecting existing assets, saving for the future, and planning for end of life.

You should also seek advice about insurance, employment rights, and state assistance programs. If possible, discuss all options with the person in your care.

Caregivers need to understand the coverage and policies of the person in their care. This includes any medical insurance, Medicare, Social Security benefits, and available private disability insurance. It also means knowing about their health insurance, coinsurance, copayments, deductibles, and covered expenses.

Caregivers also need to understand the Americans with Disabilities Act (ADA) and other laws that protect housing, transportation, recreation, and employment.

You should get help from legal and tax experts. Most communities have Legal Aid Societies. These organizations provide legal services to individuals based on income. Laws about estate planning can be confusing. This book does not cover them in detail but tells you about the tools available to you.

> **NOTE** Financial or estate planning is simply making sure that your property—no matter how little you have—goes to the person you choose as quickly and as cheaply as possible.

Financial Management Tools

Will—a legal document that spells out how money and property is to be given out after death. If a person is disabled or does not have the physical or mental abilities to tend to his or her own affairs, other legal papers are needed.

Living Trust—a legal document that names someone (a trustee) to manage a person's finances or assets. A trust includes advice on how to manage assets and when to distribute them (give them out). It can also protect assets from probate, which is a long legal process to make sure that the will is legal. Usually, the trust goes into effect if a person becomes unable to function well and is likely to make bad financial decisions.

Power of Attorney—a document that names someone to make decisions about money and property for a person who is unable to make those decision. A person should have one power of attorney for financial management and a separate power of attorney for health care.

Representative Payee—someone named by the Social Security Administration to manage a person's Social Security benefits when that person is unable to look after his or her own money and bill paying.

Conservatorship—a legal proceeding in which the court names an individual to handle another's finances when that person becomes unable to do so.

Making a will, setting up a trust, providing income, and protecting assets may involve future decisions about giving to charity, insurance policies, annuities (yearly payments), and other instruments. This kind of planning is necessary and should not be put off.

> **NOTE** Be sure to plan ahead by helping the person in your care prepare a letter of instructions. The letter should list all property and debts, location of the original will and other important documents, and names and addresses of professional advisors. It should also include funeral wishes and special instructions for giving away personal property such as furniture and jewelry.

Income Tax Considerations

In some cases, caregivers can get income tax benefits that offset their expenses as a caregiver. These tax "breaks" include claiming the person in care as a dependent and receiving a "dependent care credit." For a person who is elderly or disabled, certain tax credits also apply and some expenses are deductible.

When a Person Qualifies As a Dependent for Income Tax Purposes

A husband and wife must legally pay for each other's necessary health care, but their adult children or other relatives do not have to. However, sometimes adult children and relatives provide money or resources that will allow them to claim the person in their care as a dependent for income tax purposes.

According to the IRS, there are five tests for a person to qualify as a dependent for tax purposes:

1. The person does not earn more than a specified amount of gross income, adjusted each year to match the personal exemption. In 2007 the amount was $3,400 and in 2008 the amount is $3,500. The exemption does not apply to a child under 19, or 24 if attending school full time.

2. The taxpayer provides more than one-half of the person's support.

3. The person has one of the following relationships with the taxpayer:

- child

- brother or sister

- parent or grandparent

- aunt, uncle, niece, or nephew

- son-in-law, daughter-in-law, father-in-law, mother-in-law, brother-in-law, sister-in-law

- a descendant of a child (grandchild, great-grandchild)

- stepchild, stepbrother, stepsister, or stepparent

OR

- any person who lives in the taxpayer's home during the entire tax year and is a member of the taxpayer's household.

4. The person did not file a joint return with a spouse.

5. The person is a citizen, national, or resident of the United States, or a resident of Canada or Mexico at some time during the calendar year, or an alien child adopted by and living with a U.S. citizen.

Tax Credit for Those Who Are Elderly or Disabled

A tax credit may be available to persons who are 65 or over. It may be available to those who are permanently or totally disabled. Special rules apply for figuring out the amount of the credit. See IRS Schedule R (Form 1040) or Schedule 3 (Form 1040A).

Some life insurance policies provide tax-free benefits (accelerated death benefits), where the benefits are paid before death. Check with the life insurance company for details.

What Can Be Deducted for Income Tax Purposes

If a person can be claimed as a dependent and the caregiver itemizes, the caregiver may include medical expenses for the dependent on the caregiver's schedule of itemized deductions. If all medical expenses of the caregiver exceed 7.5% of the adjusted gross income, a deduction will be allowed.

Other deductible medical expenses are:

- improvements and additions to the home that are made for medical care purposes. (These are deductible only to the extent that they exceed the value added to the house. The entire cost of an improvement that does not increase the value of the property is deductible.)

- expenses of a dog for the blind or deaf.

- lodging while away from home for (and essential to) medical care. (The deductible expenses cannot exceed $50 per person per night. Meals are not deductible.)

- medical insurance (including premiums paid for Medicare Part B under the Social Security Act relating to supplementary medical insurance for the aged).

- long-term-care insurance premiums (subject to limitations).

- nursing homes. (The entire cost of maintenance, including meals and lodging, is deductible if the person is in a nursing home because he or she has a physical condition that requires the medical care provided.)

- transportation costs for medical care, whether around the corner or across the country. (To determine the amounts, use the actual expenses for airfare, gas, etc. If you choose, instead you may use the standard deduction of twenty-two cents per mile.)

See your tax preparer for rules about your exact situation.

STORING DOCUMENTS

Store—Death certificates, military records, tax returns for the last six years, pension documents

Keep in the safe-deposit box—Original will, deeds, passport, stock and bond certificates, birth and marriage certificates, insurance policies

Keep at home—a copy of the will that is in the safe deposit box

Throw out—expired insurance policies, checks that are more than one year old and are not tax-related

Funeral Expenses

Funeral expenses are not usually deducted for income tax purposes but are deducted if an estate tax return is filed.

Year-End Tax Tips for Family Caregivers

As early as possible, consider the following money-saving strategies and, if appropriate, discuss them with the person in your care.

- Pay or charge medical expenses in the year when the deduction will result in a benefit. Consider "bunching" medical deductions in one year (for example, buy January's prescription drugs in December).

- See if you qualify as head of household on the tax form.

- Consider transferring, to a beneficiary, title to the property that belongs to the person in your care. This makes sense when the beneficiary could claim expenses, such as real estate taxes, that the person in care could not claim because of a low income level.

- Determine who should pay medical bills by figuring out who will receive a tax deduction from the payment.

- Before selling assets to care for a parent, consider the tax that will have to be paid on the sale. Decide which assets have a high basis or a low basis (original purchase price), because capital gains should be kept low. Consider gifting first to the parent and having the parent sell at a lower tax rate.

- Consider giving property of the person in your care to a charity—and doing so in a way that provides a higher income each year than he or she would receive from interest on an investment.

TRACKING TAX-RELATED EXPENSES
- Use a file box for storage.

- Set up a separate accordion-style folder with tabs for each doctor, lab, or hospital and medicines.

- Keep all bills in the proper folder filed by month.

- Note the check number, date, and amount paid on each bill. (To keep better records, pay medical bills by check and not by credit card.)

- Keep a daily diary of cash expenses, mileage, and other travel costs for medical visits. Hand-held-devices such as a Palm Pilot are useful for keeping this information.

Social Security Benefits

The Social Security Administration runs two federal disability retirement programs: Social Security Disability Insurance (SSDI) and Supplemental Security Income (SSI). SSDI is an insurance program that is funded by taxes from employees and employers. SSI is an assistance program for people with low incomes. The medical requirements and disability standards are the same.

Social Security considers a person disabled when he or she is unable to perform a paid job for which he or she is suited and the disability is expected to last for 12 months.

As a result of 2002 federal tax laws, people over 65 have no limits on the amount they can earn and still receive Social Security benefits. Call the Social Security Administration (1-800-772-1213) to get a report of your benefits record.

Understanding Social Security

- Retirement checks are loosely tied to how much a person paid into the system.

- Social Security provides the money for people who become disabled; once on disability for two years, one would be eligible for Medicare benefits. If the person receiving Social Security dies, it also takes care of that person's spouse and children. The death benefit is $255.

- In 2007, Social Security typically pays $1044 a month for the average retired worker.

- Social Security, personal savings, and employer pensions together provide financial support in old age.

NOTE Name the personal representative as co-renter of the safe deposit box if the person in your care does not have a spouse or close relative. This will make it easier to get into the safe deposit box after death

Medicaid Guidelines

The cost of nursing home care is high and can easily wipe out a couple's savings even if only one person is in a nursing home.

Currently, Medicaid rules allow a person:

- to keep a home if he or she plans to return there or if it is lived in by a spouse or a disabled or minor child

- to have a maximum individual income (which varies state to state), including pension payments and Social Security

- to have a prepaid funeral fund of $1,500

- to have a bank account of no more than $2,000

General Points Regarding Asset Transfers

- Transfers must happen at least 60 months before applying to a nursing facility. (Transfers within 60 months may delay eligibility for Medicaid. Certain transfers from trusts can delay eligibility for up to 60 months.)

- A home can be transferred within 60 months if it is transferred to a spouse, a minor, or a disabled child.

- Transfers of assets to a child may be risky if the child will not be able or willing to help the parent if extra money is needed.

- A trust may be a better option because the money is still available for the parents' needs.

- If a person sets up a special-needs trust for himself, the assets must still be spent down to qualify for Medicaid payment for nursing home care.

- Among the penalties for people who transfer assets for less than fair market value to qualify for Medicaid is a $10,000 fine and up to a year in prison.

- The healthy spouse of a person who applies for Medicaid may retain some income and resources. Each case is assessed after the applicant becomes eligible for Medicaid.

- The most individual income a person can have and still get Medicaid varies from state to state. The rules can be tricky, so seek the advice of an attorney.

Employment Planning

Employment planning and retirement tips are very important. There are many issues to look into once the care receiver can no longer work. You will need to look at sick leave, short-term disability insurance, and the Family Medical Leave Act. When the person in your care decides to stop working, you will need to look into options for medical coverage. Applying for long-term disability benefits and Social Security can take a lot of time. You will need to find out what you can do while waiting for these new benefits.

You will also need to think about tapping into other sources of income once you decide to leave work: applying for Social Security or veterans benefits; the cash value of life insurance, long-term-care insurance; personal property, real estate, and mortgage insurance.

Abuse by Financial Advisors

Aggressive marketing to the elderly is becoming increasingly common. Although seminars for estate planning can provide useful information, they are often selling something and therefore do not offer an unbiased assessment of what a person may need. Help the person in your care avoid financial planners who may also be stock brokers or insurance agents. Before selecting a financial planner, one should always:

- Check with the local Area Agency on Aging and other agencies that work with the elderly for a list of referrals.

- Interview the financial planner and check his or her credentials (law, accounting degrees, continuing education in financial planning for the retired).

- Find out what the financial advisor will gain from your business in fee and commission income.

- Take this information into account before deciding to buy.

- Ask for the fees in writing.

- Ask if local law requires that any comparisons of plans be provided.

- Ask if the advisor is registered with the Securities and Exchange Commission.

Neither the authors nor the publisher are engaged in providing legal or tax services. This *Guide* is for general information only. In order to learn more about these matters, consult a CPA, attorney, or other professional advisor.

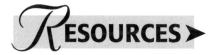

AARP Tax-Aide
www.aarp.org/taxaide/home.htm (for a listing of site locations)
(888) 227-7669
Call 24 hours a day, 7 days a week to find a site near you. Provides free help on federal, state and local tax returns to middle- and low-income persons aged 60 years and older; also

provides online counselors at the Web site. This program also accepts volunteers.

Certified Financial Planners Board of Standards
(800) 487-1497; (303) 830-7500; (888) 237-6275
www.cfp-board.org
This organization will provide information on whether a planner is certified, how long he or she has been certified, and if any disciplinary action has ever been taken.

Financial Planning Association
Suite 400, 4100 E. Mississippi Ave.
Denver, CO 80246-3053
(800) 322-4237
Fax (404) 845-3660
www.fpanet.org
Web site provides a list and backgrounds of certified financial planners in your region and a helpful free pamphlet, Selecting a Qualified Financial Planning Professional, which lists questions you should ask a financial planner before hiring him or her.

IRS Web Site
(800) 829-3676 for publications; (800) 829-1040 for answers to tax questions
www.irs.gov
The Web site provides tax forms. Form 559 is for survivors, and Form 524 is for those who are elderly or disabled.

National Association of Personal Financial Advisors
www.napfa.org

Older Women's League
3300 N. Fairfax Drive, Suite 218
Arlington, VA 22201
(800) 825-3695; (703) 812-7990
Fax (703) 812-0687
www.owl-national.org

Paralyzed Veterans of America
www.pva.org
Keys to Managed Care: A Guide for People with Physical Disabilities is available at the Web site.

Social Security Administration
(800) 772-1213
www.socialsecurity.gov
Provides a personal report on a person's Social Security record.

Society of Financial Service Professionals
www.financialpro.org

If you don't have home access to the Internet, ask your local library to help you locate any Web site.

Preparing the Home

Preparing the Home

*A*dapting the home for a person who is partially or fully disabled can be a difficult process or a simple process. In general, the more adaptations (changes) that can be made early on—with a view toward future needs—the easier life will be for everyone concerned. Few caregivers can afford to remodel a home totally. Yet, it is important for readers to be aware of the "ideal" as they plan the changes that make sense for their situations.

Here we present suggestions—from architects who specialize in elder care housing, occupational therapists, and others—for setting up the best home care conditions.

Safety, Safety, Safety

The main concern in any home is safety. Accidents can happen, but with a little planning can be prevented. Take a close look at the home where you will provide care. You may want to ask a relative or friend to look at it with you to make sure you haven't overlooked any safety hazards.

> **NOTE** Leave a blanket, pillow, and phone on the floor; however, not in the flow of foot traffic. In case of a fall, the person in your care can stay warm and call for help. A care receiver who spends time alone should always have a cell phone with him.

As you plan for safety in the home, think about what you will need now and what you will need in the future. For example, people with liver disease often have problems with blood clotting and therefore furniture should be arranged to avoid bumps and bruises. Sharp corners need to be padded.

As you make changes to the home, don't forget your own comfort and ease. Making life easier for yourself means you will have more time to provide care or to rest. In the long run, this will improve the overall setting for care.

The Home Setting

Safety

For the safest home, follow as many of these steps as possible:

- Remove any furniture that is not needed.

- Place the remaining furniture so that there is enough space for a walker or wheelchair. This will avoid the need to move around coffee tables and other barriers. Move any low tables that are in the way.

- Once the person in your care has gotten used to where the furniture is, do not change it.

- Make sure furniture will not move if it is leaned on.

- Make sure the armrests of a favorite chair are long enough to help the person get up and down.

- Add cushioning to sharp corners on furniture, cabinets, and vanities.

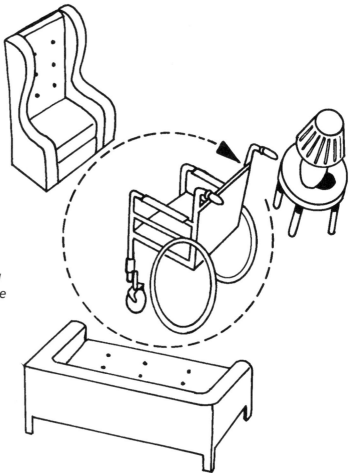

To accommodate a wheelchair, arrange furniture 5½ feet a part.

- Have a carpenter install railings in places where a person might need extra support. (Using a carpenter can ensure that railings can bear a person's full weight and will not give way.)

- Place masking or colored tape on glass doors and picture windows.

- Use automatic night-lights in the rooms used by the person in your care.

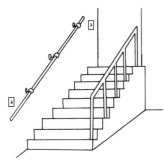

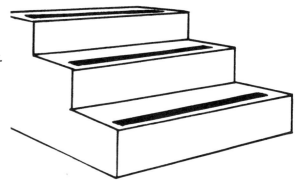

▶ *Place nonskid tape on the edges of steps.*

▲ *Always provide railings along stairways. When possible, extend the handrailpast the bottom and top step*

- Clear fire-escape routes.

- Provide smoke alarms on every floor and outside every bedroom.

- Place a fire extinguisher in the kitchen.

- Think about using monitors and intercoms.

- Place nonskid tape on the edges of stairs (and consider painting the edge of the first and last step a different color from the floor).

- It is easier to walk on thin-pile carpet than on thick pile. Avoid busy patterns.

- Be sure stairs have even surfaces with no metal strips or rubber mats to cause tripping.

- Remove all hazards that might lead to tripping.

- Tape or tack electrical and telephone cords to walls.

- Adjust or remove rapidly closing doors.

- Place protective screens on fireplaces.

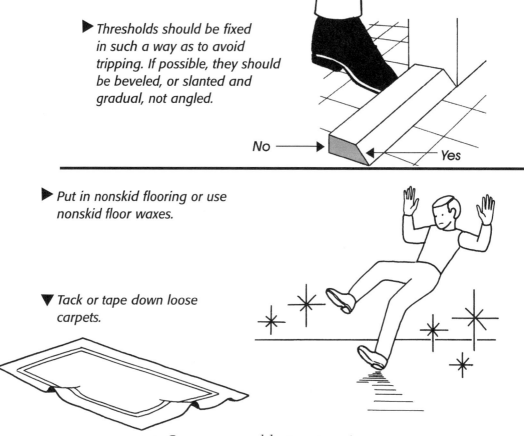

▶ *Thresholds should be fixed in such a way as to avoid tripping. If possible, they should be beveled, or slanted and gradual, not angled.*

No ⟶   ⟵ Yes

▶ *Put in nonskid flooring or use nonskid floor waxes.*

▼ *Tack or tape down loose carpets.*

- Cover exposed hot-water pipes.

- Provide enough no-glare lighting—indirect is best.

- Place light switches next to room entrances so the lights can be turned on before entering a room. Consider "clap-on" lamps beside the bed.

- Use 100 to 200–watt lightbulbs for close-up activities (but make sure lamps can handle the extra wattage).

- Plan for extra outdoor lighting for good nighttime visibility, especially on stairs and walkways.

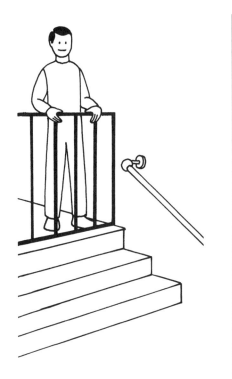

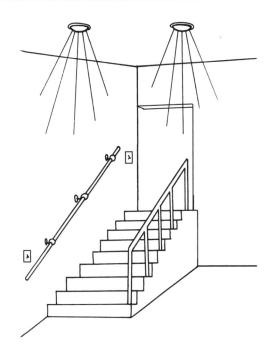

▲ *Be sure steps are well lighted with light switches at both the top and bottom of the stairs.*

▲ *A safety gate at the top of stairs can prevent falls.*

- If possible, install a carbon monoxide (CO) detector that sounds an alarm when dangerous levels of CO are reached. Call the **American Lung Association** (800) LUNG USA, for details.

- Work out an emergency escape plan in case of fire.

NOTE If the person in your care is on life-support equipment, install a backup electrical power system and have a plan of action in case the power goes out.

Comfort and Convenience

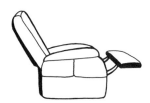

▲ *Think about getting a power-assisted recliner that allows the power-assist feature to be turned off.*

- For persons who are frail or wheelchair-bound, put in automatic door openers.

- For a person with a wheelchair or a walker, allow at least 18–24″ clearance from the door on landings.

- Plan to leave enough space (a minimum of 32″ clear) for moving a hospital bed and wheelchair through doorways.

▶ *Install entry ramps. Rails can be added for more safety.*

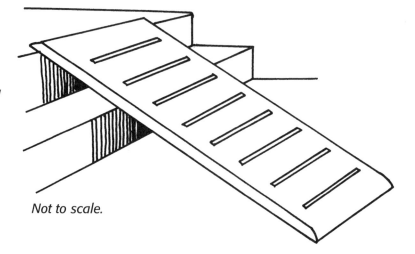

Not to scale.

NOTE If you are redoing or building a new two-story house, have the contractor frame in the shell of the elevator and then add the elevator unit later when needed. Use the space as a closet for now.

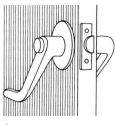

▲ Lever handle

- To widen doorways, remove the molding and replace regular door hinges with offset hinges. Whenever possible, remove doors.

- Put lever-type handles on all doors.

- If a person who is disabled must be moved from one story to another, install a stair elevator.

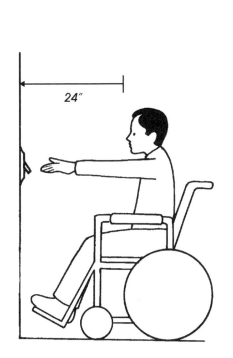
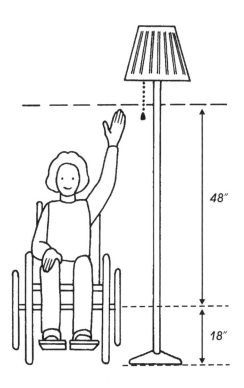

▲ *A person can reach forward about 24" from a seated position. Between18" and 48" from the floor is the ideal position for light switches, telephones, and mail boxes.*

The Bathroom

Many accidents happen in bathrooms, so check the safety of the bathroom that you will use for home care.

Safety

▶ *Install grab bars beside the toilet, along the edge of the sink, and in the tub and the shower according to the needs of each person.*

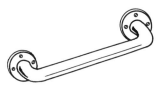

▶ *Five-inch door pulls or utility handles can be put on door frames and window sills.*

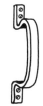

- Cover all sharp edges with rubber cushioning.

- Put lights in the medicine cabinets so mistakes are not made when taking medicine.

- Remove locks on bathroom doors.

- Use nonskid safety strips or a nonslip bath mat in the tub or shower.

- Think about putting a grab rail on the edge of the vanity. (Do not use a towel bar.)

- Remove glass shower doors or replace them with unbreakable plastic.

- Use only electrical appliances with a ground fault interrupted (GFI) feature.

- Install GFI electrical outlets.

- Set the hot water thermostat below 120° F.

- Use faucets that mix hot and cold water, or paint hot water knobs/faucets red.

- Insulate (cover) hot water pipes to prevent burns.

- Put in toilet guard rails or provide a portable toilet seat with built-in rails. (See p. 144)

Comfort and Convenience

- If possible, the bathroom should be in a straight path from the bedroom of the person in your care.

- Put in a ceiling heat lamp.

- Place a telephone near the toilet.

- Provide soap-on-a-rope or put a bar of soap in the toe of a nylon stocking and tie it to the grab bar.

- Place toilet paper within easy reach.

- Try to provide enough space for two people at the bathroom sink.

- If possible, have the sink 32″–34″ from the floor.

- Use levers instead of handles on faucets.

- Provide an elevated (raised) toilet seat.

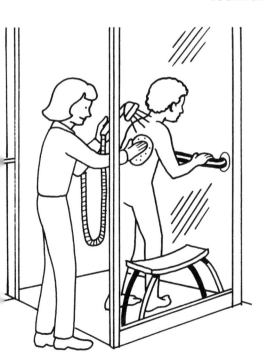

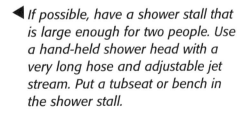

◀ If possible, have a shower stall that is large enough for two people. Use a hand-held shower head with a very long hose and adjustable jet stream. Put a tubseat or bench in the shower stall.

The Kitchen

Many of the following suggestions are made to fit the needs of people who are handicapped. Some of these may help liver patients depending on their health situation.

Safety

- Use an electric teakettle.

- Set the water-heater temperature at 120° F.

- Use a single-lever faucet that can balance water temperature.

- Provide an area away from the knife drawer and the stove where the person in your care can help prepare food.

- Use a microwave oven whenever possible (but not if a person with a pacemaker is present).

- Ask the gas company to modify your stove to provide a gas odor that is strong enough to alert you if the pilot light goes out.

- If possible, have the range controls on the front of the stove.

- Provide a step stool, never a chair, to reach high shelves.

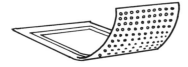

▲ *Cover the floor with a nonslip surface or use a nonskid mat near the sink, where it may be wet.*

Comfort and Convenience

- Use adjustable-height chairs with locking casters.

- Install a Lazy Susan® (swivel plate) in corner cabinets.

- Set up cabinets to reduce bending and reaching.

- Put in a storage wall rather than upper cabinets.

- For easy access, replace drawer knobs with handles.

▶ Use "reachers"—devices for reaching objects in high or low places without stretching, bending, or standing on a stool.

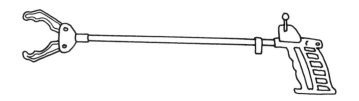

▶ A cutting board placed over a drawer provides an easy-to-reach surface for a person in a wheelchair.

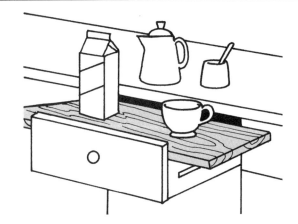

- Place a wire rack on the counter to reduce back strain from reaching dishes.

- Adapt one counter for wheelchair access as pictured above.

- Remove doors under the sink to allow for wheelchair access; also cover exposed pipes.

- Create different counter heights by putting in folding or pull-out surfaces.

- If bending is difficult, consider a wall oven.

- Use suspension systems for heavy drawers.

- Put pullout shelves in cabinets.

- If possible, use a fridge that has the freezer on the bottom.

- Prop the front of the fridge so that the door closes by itself. (If necessary, reverse the way the door swings.)

The Bedroom

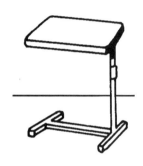

▲ *Provide an adjustable over-the-bed table like the ones used to serve meals in hospital rooms.*

Ideally, provide three bedrooms—one for the person in care, one for yourself, and one for the home health aide. Also

- Put in a monitor to listen to activity in the room of the person in your care. (Most are inexpensive and are portable.)

- Make the bedroom bright and cheerful.

- Make sure enough heat (65°F at night) and fresh air are available.

- Provide a firm mattress.

- Provide TV and radio.

- Think about having a fish tank for fun and relaxation.

- Use throwaway pads to protect furniture.

- Install blinds or shades that darken the room.

- Place closet rods 48″ from the floor.

- Provide a chair for dressing.

- Keep a flashlight at the bedside table.

- Provide a bedside commode with a 4″ foam pad on the seat for comfort if needed.

- Hang a bulletin board with pictures of family and friends where it can be easily seen.

- Provide a sturdy chair or table next to the bed for help getting in and out of bed.

- Make the bed 22″ high and place it securely against a wall. Or use lockable wheels. This will allow the person to get up and down safely.

- Use blocks to raise a bed's height, but be sure to make them steady so they don't move.

▶ *Bedside commode and bed with trapeze bar.*

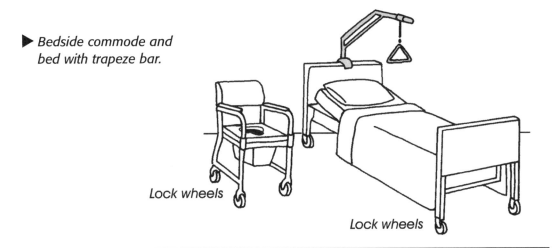

Lock wheels

Lock wheels

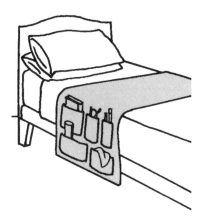

▲ *Make a bed organizer to hold facial tissues, lotion, and other items needed at the bedside. Do this by attaching pockets to a large piece of fabric spread across the bed.*

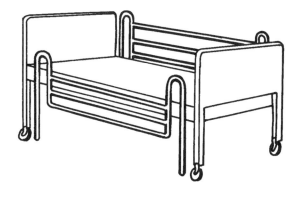

▲ *If all the care is at the bedside, consider a hospital bed. This will be helpful for both you and the person in your care.*

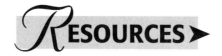

RESOURCES

AARP
601 E Street, NW
Washington, DC 20049
(800) 424-3410
www.aarp.org
Call or write for the booklet, The Do-Able, Renewable Home. Members can receive one copy at no charge.

Center for Universal Design
North Carolina State University
Box 8613
Raleigh, NC 27695-8613
(800) 647-6777; (919) 515-3082 (V/TTY)
Fax: (919) 515-3023
www.design.ncsu.edu\cud
E-mail: cud@ncsu.edu
Established by the National Institute on Disability and Rehabilitation Research (NIDRR) to improve the quality and availability of housing for people with disabilities. Services include information, referral service, training and education, technical design assistance, and publications.

Metropolitan Center for Independent Living, Inc. (MCIL)
1600 University Avenue West, Suite 16
St. Paul, MN 55104-3825
(651) 603-2029
www.wheelchairramp.org
E-mail: jimwi@mcil-mn.org
Web site features How to Build Wheelchair Ramps for Homes, an online manual for the design and construction of wheelchair ramps.

National Association of Home Builders Research Center
(800) 638-8556; (301) 249-4000
www.nahbrc.org
Call for its book A Comprehensive Approach to Retrofitting Houses for a Lifetime, $15 plus postage and handling.

National Institute for Rehabilitation Engineering
P.O. Box 1088
Hewett, NJ 07421
(800) 736-2216; (973) 853-6585 Fax (928) 832-2894
www.theoffice.net/nire
E-mail: nire@theoffice.net

Paralyzed Veterans of America
801 18th Street NW
Washington, DC 20006-3517
(800) 424-8200
www.pva.org
Not just for veterans, not just for paralysis. Ask for the Architecture Program.

Check with local police to find out if they manage a **Senior Locks Program**. This program can install deadbolt locks and other security devices for homeowners 55 and older who meet federal income guidelines.

Part Two: Day by Day

Setting Up a Plan of Care

Setting Up a Plan of Care

A plan of care is a daily record of the care and treatment a person needs after a hospital stay. The plan helps you and the person in your care with caregiving tasks.

When a person leaves a hospital, the discharge planner provides the caregiver with a copy of the doctor's orders and a brief set of instructions for care. The discharge planner also works with a home health care agency to send a nurse to help the caregiver. The nurse will evaluate the person in care's needs for equipment, personal care, help with shots or medication, etc. The nurse will also work with the entire health care team (including you as the caregiver, a physical therapist, and other specialists) to develop a detailed plan of care.

The plan of care includes the following information:

- *diagnosis (the nature of the disease)*

- *medications*

- *functional limitations (what the person can and cannot do)*

- *special diet*

- *detailed care instructions and comments*

- *services the home health care agency provides*

The information is presented in a certain order so that the process of care is repeated over and over until it becomes routine. When the plan is kept up to date, it provides a clear record of events that helps solve problems and avoid them.

With a plan, you don't have to rely on your memory. It also allows another person to take over respite care or take your place entirely without too much trouble.

Some of the things you may have to watch and record are

- *skin color, warmth, and tone (dryness, firmness, etc.)*

- *breathing, temperature, pulse, and blood pressure*

- *circulation (dark red or blue spots on the legs or feet)*

- *fingernails and toenails (any unusual conditions)*

- *mobility (ability to move around)*

- *swelling of the hands, ankles, and the abdomen*

- *appetite*

- *body posture (relaxed, twisted, or stiff)*

- *bowel and bladder function (unusual changes)*

- *cognitve function - watch for confusion*

Tip

Watch out for stool and urine color changes. For example, dark black and bright red stool may indicate bleeding, and dark urine may be a sign of dehydration and worsening liver disease.

Recording the Plan of Care

Use a loose-leaf notebook to record the plan of care. Put the doctor's instructions on the inside front cover (always keep the originals).

Recording and Managing Medications

Always be sure that the person in your care takes the medication exactly as prescribed. Keep an accurate list of these medications and when they should be taken.

Never make any changes to these medications without talking to the specialist first. However, because everyone's treatment needs are different, the specialist may want to try changing the amount or timing of drugs, within certain limits. If you are worried or have any questions, don't be afraid to ask your doctor or pharmacist for advice.

People who have serious health problems often take a large number of medications at many different times of the day. It is essential to have a careful system for keeping track of medications:

- when medications should be given

- how they should be given

- when they were actually given

The following sample of a weekly medication schedule is a good model to follow. Be sure to fill in the times when (A.M. and P.M.) medications actually were given, and have each caregiver initial them.

Weekly Medication Schedule (Sample Form)

Medication	Date/Time/Initials						
Name, dose, frequency, with or without food	Sat.	Sun.	Mon.	Tues.	Wed.	Thurs.	Fri.
Example							
Lactulose 30 cc three times per day and titrate to 3–4 pudding-like bowel movements per day							
Lasix 40 mg 1x daily a.m.							
Aldactone 50 mg 1x daily							
Propranolol 10 mg 3X daily							

As you finish your own schedule, be sure to record information from the label of each prescription, including

- days of the week when each medicine must be taken

- number of times per day

- time of day

- whether the medicine is to be taken with or without food

- how much water should be taken with the medicine

Also make a note to yourself about any warnings (for example, "Don't take this medicine with food/milk OR do not take it with another medicine) and possible side effects (dizziness, confusion, headache, etc.).

> **Tip**
>
> For people with end-stage liver disease, dehydration can lead to worsening confusion, therefore it is important to make sure the person in care does not develop diarrhea from taking lactulose.

NOTE Labels may contain the following abbreviations that you should be aware of:

HS—hour of sleep (medication time)
BID—give the medicine 2 times per day (approximately 8 am and 8 pm)
TID—give the medicine 3 times per day (approximately 9 am, 1 pm, 6 pm)
QID—give the medicine 4 times per day (approximately 9 am, 1 pm, 5 pm, 9 pm)
QAC—give the medication before each meal

Other Cautions

- Never crush drugs without talking to the doctor or pharmacist first. If the person in your care has trouble swallowing medication, ask the doctor if there is another way it can be taken. (See *Using the Health Care Team Effectively,* p. 41.)

- If the person in your care will take the medicine without your help, ask the pharmacist to use easy-open caps on prescription bottles.

- Do not store medicine that will be taken internally (swallowed) in the same cabinet with medicine that will be used externally (lotions, salves, creams, etc.).

- Keep a magnifying glass near the medicine cabinet for reading small print.

- Store most medicine in a cool, dry place—usually not the bathroom. Some may require refrigeration

- Remove the cotton from each bottle so that moisture is not drawn in.

- Check with your pharmacist about disposal options for expired medications in your area. Dispose of needles in the sharp containers and return to the appropriate agency (local pharmacy, doctor's office, local hospital etc.).

- Check the expiration dates on all the medication bottles. Contact the prescribing physician if the medication has expired to see if the person in your care still needs the medication.

- Check for duplicate medications. Remember that the person in your care may have two different doctors prescribing the same medications either at the same dose or different doses. Clarify any differences with the prescribing physician first.

- If childproof containers are too hard to open, ask the pharmacist for containers that are not childproof.

EMERGENCY PREPAREDNESS
Let the local fire station and ambulance company know that a person with disabilities lives at your address. They will have the information on hand and can respond quickly.

Emergency Information

Have this information posted near telephones or on the refrigerator, where it can be used by anyone in the household in case of emergency.

Personal Information

Name _____ Date of Birth _____

Address _____

Phone _____

SS # _____ Supplemental Insurance # _____

Medicaid # _____ Medicare # _____

Current Medications: _____

_____

Exact Location of Do Not Resuscitate Order: _____

Emergency Numbers

Fire _____ Police _____

Ambulance _____ Hospital _____

Doctor _____

Drugstore _____ Open Till _____ Delivers _____

Family Caregiver Work Number _____

Alternate Caregiver _____

Home Health Care Agency _____

Medicare Toll Free Number _____

Insurance _____

Medical Equipment Company _____

Poison Control _____

Friend _____

Neighbor _____ Relative _____

Clergy/Rabbi _____

Transport Number _____ Meals-on-Wheels _____

Shopping Assistance _____

Directions for Driving to the House _____

_____

_____

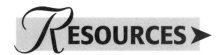

RESOURCES ➤

Drug Interaction Checker
www.medscape.com/drugchecker

General Caregiving Books

Always on Call: When Illness Turns Families into Caregivers, by Carol Levine (Ed.).
United Hospital Fund, 2000.

The Complete Eldercare Planner, by Joy Loverde.
Three Rivers Press, 2000.

How to Avoid Caregiver Burnout

How to Avoid Caregiver Burnout

*P*roviding emotional support and physical care to an ill person can be deeply satisfying, but it can be upsetting. Sometimes it is simply more than one person can handle. The strain of balancing a job, a family, more work in the home, and the care of someone may lead you to feel like a martyr or angry and guilty. Most people with end-stage liver disease are able to care for themselves (ADL). So it is not highly physically demanding for the caregiver. However, some can be very weak and wheelchair bound where physical care is needed.

One of the biggest mistakes caregivers make is thinking that they can—and should—do everything by themselves. The best way to avoid burnout is to have the practical and emotional support of other people. Sharing concerns with others not only relieves stress, but also can give you a new slant on problems.

Because people with end-stage liver disease who are waiting for liver transplant wait for a long time and there is no guarantee that they will get a liver transplant, they can die while waiting. They may be mild to moderately sick for a long time, but not sick enough to get a liver transplant. The progression varies and there is a lot of uncertainty, which can increase anxiety and frustration in patients and caregivers. This is something very unique to liver transplant since the transplant does not happen on a "first-come first-served" basis. It is important to have support and open communication to deal with this.

Negative Emotions That May Arise in You

The challenges of the caregiver role may sometimes make you feel bad about yourself. If you are a perfectionist, you'll never do it perfectly. If you're angry, you'll find plenty of excuses to be mad. If you have feelings of inadequacy, they'll definitely come up. Impatience, depression, hostility—if these emotions challenged you before, they're sure to arise in this situation.

Guilt Is Crippling

Opportunities for guilt can come up often in caregiving. Even if you are doing it perfectly, you can easily convince yourself that you're not doing enough. People who are waiting for liver transplant can get much worse suddenly. The caregiver may feel guilty about "not doing enough" to prevent that. But it is important to understand that the sudden deterioration is part of the nature of the disease and sometimes cannot be prevented. To combat this tendency, *at least once a day, every day*, remind yourself :

- about how you are helping the person in your care

- when you don't do things perfectly, you are doing them with love

- you have grown in skill and compassion

Depression Is Dangerous

Just as depression endangers your care receiver's recovery, it also endangers your health and well-being. Depression increases your risk in every major disease category, particularly cardiovascular disease.

Symptoms of Depression

Here are the symptoms:

- persistent sad, anxious or "empty" mood

- feelings of hopelessness, pessimism

- feelings of guilt, worthlessness, helplessness

- loss of interest or pleasure in hobbies and activities that were once enjoyed, including sex

119

- decreased energy, fatigue, being "slowed down"
- difficulty concentrating, remembering, making decisions
- insomnia, early-morning awakening, or oversleeping
- appetite and/or weight changes
- thoughts of death or suicide, or suicidal attempts
- restlessness, irritability

If you have five or more of these symptoms for longer than two weeks, depression may be the cause. Talk to a physician, psychiatrist, or psychologist about treatment options. The most effective treatment combines medication with talking therapy.

- Claim time for yourself and make sure you use it; otherwise, you will burn out and the person in your care will suffer.

- Make and keep doctor's appointments for yourself; otherwise, when you get sick, everyone will suffer.

- Join a caregiver support group; otherwise, you and the person in your care will suffer isolation.

- Take advantage of respite care opportunities, otherwise, when you break down the person in your care will suffer.

Anger

It is easy to feel victimized in this situation; you are caught up in someone else's illness. The natural response is anger. Unfortunately, that is not a helpful response. Unleashing anger on the person in your care never helps.

On the other hand, it is not good for you to stuff those feelings. There are definite consequences to your health and well-being. Try these outlets:

- Caregiver support groups provide a place where you can vent feelings. Everyone there understands; no one will make you feel guilty. Members will often offer effective, real-world solutions. Scientific evidence indicates caregivers who participate in support groups are better able to deal with the situation.

- Make an appointment with a therapist or family counselor or clergyperson. If possible, make two appointments: one for you alone and one for you and the person in your care.

- Keep a journal of your feelings.

- Remember, people who have lost control may try to regain it by controlling what they can, which may be their caregivers.

- Separate the person from the condition. The illness, not the person in your care, is responsible for the difficulties and challenges that you both are facing. Don't blame the care receiver for the situation you are in.

- Set and enforce limits on how many non-essential needs you will fill per hour, such as pouring water or changing channels. Non-emergency care does not have to be handled immediately.

Tip

Sometimes it is necessary to tell the person in your care how you are feeling, but it is important not to accuse him personally. Saying "You make me feel angry" may worsen the situation. Instead say, "Just as I am trying to understand what you are going through, please try to understand what I am going through with you."

Emotional Burdens

You may think you are the only one to face these problems, but you are not alone. Every caregiver faces—

- the need to hide his or her grief

- fear of the future

- worries about money

- having less ability to solve problems

Dependency and Isolation

Fears of dependency and loneliness, or isolation, are common in families of those who are ill. The person needing care can become more and more dependent on the one who is providing it. At the same time, the caregiver needs others for respite and support. Many caregivers are ashamed about needing help, so they don't ask for it. Those caregivers who are able to develop personal and social support have a greater sense of well-being.

 Men who are caregivers face special problems. Often they are not used to doing daily chores around the house. They also lose the emotional support of the spouse who is ill and must now be her support. It is especially important for men to seek out a support system.

Knowing When to Seek Help

"Why doesn't anyone ask how I am doing?" It is easy to feel invisible, as if no one can see you. Everyone's attention is on the person with the illness, and they don't seem to understand what the caregiver is going through. Many caregivers say that nobody even asks how they're doing. Mental health experts say it's not wise to let feelings of neglect build up. Caregivers need to speak up and tell other people what they need and how they feel.

Support groups, religious or spiritual advisors, or mental health counselors can teach you new and positive ways to express your own need for help.

Seek out professional help when you:

- are using more alcohol than usual to relax

- are using too many prescription medications

- have physical symptoms such as skin rashes, backaches, or a cold or flu that won't go away

- are unable to think clearly or focus

- feel tired and don't want to do anything

- feel keyed up and on edge

- feel sad all the time

- feel intense fear and anxiety

- feel worthless and guilty

- are depressed for two weeks or more

- are having thoughts of suicide

- have become or are thinking about becoming physically violent toward the person you are caring for

When Hostility Builds to the Breaking Point

Anger is a common emotion for caregivers and for the person being cared for. The situation feels—and is—unfair. Both may say hurtful words during a difficult task. Someone may slam a door during a disagreement. Shouting sometimes replaces conversation. Anger and frustration must be addressed and healthy outlets found as a way to let off steam. If they are not, angry situations can become physically or emotionally abusive. (📖 See ***Abuse,*** p. 164)

You can control your emotions by letting go of anger and frustration in a safe way.

- Take a walk to cool down.

- Write your thoughts in a journal.

- Go to a private corner and take out your anger on a big pillow.

Checklist **Dealing with Physical and Emotional Burdens**

✓ Do not allow the person in your care to take unfair advantage of you by being overly demanding.

✓ Live one day at a time.

✓ List priorities, decide what to leave undone, and think of ways to make the work easier.

✓ When doing a long, boring care task, use the time to relax or listen to music.

✓ Find time for regular exercise to increase your energy (even if you only stretch in place).

✓ Focus on getting relaxing sleep rather than more sleep.

✓ Take several short rests in order to get enough sleep.

✓ Set aside time for prayer or reflection.

✓ Practice deep breathing and learn to meditate to empty your mind of all troubles.

✓ Allow your self-esteem to rise because you have discovered hidden skills and talents.

✓ Realize your own limitations and accept them.

✓ Make sure your goals are realistic—you may be unable to do everything you could do before.

✓ Keep your eating habits balanced—do not fall into a toast-and-tea habit.

✓ *Take time for yourself.*

✓ *Treat yourself to a massage.*

✓ *Keep up with outside friends and activities.*

✓ *Spread the word that you would welcome some help, and allow friends to help with respite care.*

✓ *Delegate (assign) jobs to others. Keep a list of tasks you need to have done and assign specific ones when people offer to help.*

✓ *Share your concerns with a friend.*

✓ *Join a support group, or start one (to share ideas and resources).*

✓ *Use respite care when needed.*

✓ *Express yourself openly and honestly with people you feel should be doing more to help.*

✓ *When you visit your own doctor, be sure to explain your caregiving responsibilities, not just your symptoms.*

✓ *Allow yourself to feel your emotions without guilt. They are natural and very human.*

✓ *Unload your anger and frustration by writing it down.*

✓ *Allow yourself to cry and sob.*

✓ *Know that you are providing a very important service to the person in your care.*

Where to Find Professional Help or Support Groups

- the community pages of the phone directory
- the local county medical society, which can provide a list of counselors, psychologists, and psychiatrists
- religious service agencies
- community health clinics
- religious and spiritual advisors
- United Way's "First Call for Help"
- a hospital's social service department
- a newspaper calendar listing of support group meetings
- parish nurses
- Area Agency on Aging

Ask for help from a counselor who is familiar with the needs of caregivers.

Self-Care for Caregivers

If you don't take care of yourself, then you won't finish the caregiving race, and the care receiver will suffer. Part of your responsibility to the person in your care is to take care of yourself.

Tip

Here's a thought to keep in mind: In the safety talk before every flight, the stewardess tells parents to put the oxygen mask on themselves first and then the child. Why? Because if the parent passes out, the child's safety is at risk.

Exercise

Even moderate exercise is beneficial because it breaks the cycle of being sedentary. And being sedentary is a risk factor for all major diseases.

Walking is easy, and if you can't walk for 30–40 minutes at a stretch, several 5–10 minute periods are enough. Exercise improves mood and physique and can be an opportunity to socialize. Find a way to make it part of your day.

Tip

If you can't join a gym, investigate the YMCA. Some larger churches often have low- or no-cost exercise classes.

Eat Right

Nutrition is critical to your well-being. Learn to read labels and avoid foods with high fat content. Monitor your portion size; for example, a proper serving of meat is about the size of a deck of playing cards.

The person in your care will almost certainly be given a dietary prescription. In cooking heart-healthy for him, you will benefit yourself and the rest of your family. (📖 See **Diet, Nutrition, and Exercise,** p. 175)

Tip

Calorie-dense foods pack a lot of calories in a small package—think chocolate. For example, 8oz of broccoli is 65 calories; 8oz of chocolate chip cookies is 1,070 calories. Fresh fruits and vegetables will typically have many fewer calories than processed foods. Canned fruit often has added sugar and salt. Cooking for the caregiver and the person in your care at the same time is more effective and often time healthier for both.

> **Tip**
>
> Most people need to eat more fruit—9 servings a day. To help you meet that goal, keep a bowl of apples, oranges, pears, bananas, and seasonal fruits on a kitchen counter and nibble on the fruit throughout the day.

> **Tip**
>
> For reliable and easy-to-understand information on nutrition; changing your diet; easy-to-follow eating plans; and quick, tasty, and healthy recipes, go to www.AmericanHeart.org. It is a free, one-stop shop for heart-healthy nutrition. Visit www.AASLD.org for dietary recommendation for liver disease patients.

Take Care of the Caregiver

Many caregivers neglect their own physical health. They ignore what is ailing them and don't take steps to avoid getting sick, such as exercising, eating a proper diet, and getting regular medical examinations.

Many caregivers do not get enough sleep at night. If sleep is regularly broken up because the person in your care needs help during the night, talk about the problems with a health care professional.

The person in your care needs a healthy caregiver. Both partners need uninterrupted sleep.

Meditation

Your journey as a caregiver will be more satisfying and less stressful if you take up a practice of daily meditation. Think of meditation as sitting still doing nothing. Here are seven easy steps:

1. Sit so your back is straight, either on a chair or a big, firm pillow.

2. As you inhale, tense your whole body—arms, legs, buttocks, fists, scrunch your face.

3. Hold 2–3 seconds.

4. Exhale and relax (repeat twice).

5. Take a deep breath, let your belly expand.

6. Exhale and relax (repeat twice).

7. Breathe normally and observe your thoughts for five minutes.

Tip

Most people fail at meditation because they think meditation means clearing your mind of thoughts. Instead of emptying your mind of thoughts, observe them. There are no "right" thoughts to think. Don't focus on any of your thoughts and don't fight with any of them. An easy way to do that is to label each one as it bubbles up—sad thought, happy thought, angry thought, depressed thought, to-do list thought—and let it go and then label the next one that appears.

Tip

A kitchen timer will alert you to five minutes.

It is not important how long you sit with your eyes closed and observe your thoughts—5 minutes will do, especially to start. What makes meditation effective at reducing stress is the *practice* **of meditation, doing it every day. You can do it before the person in your care wakes up or after she goes to bed or is taking a nap. It's only 5 or 10 minutes, but the cumulative effect over just a few weeks is noticeable. (For more on meditation, visit www.mycalmspace.com.)**

Plan for the Long Term: Winning the Caregiving Race

Most people jump into caregiving as if it were a sprint. They think they can and must do everything themselves. You may be able to do that for a few weeks or even months, but the average caregiver spends more than few years in that role—no one can sprint for that long.

Instead of a sprint, treat caregiving as a marathon—for which you have not trained—and pace yourself accordingly from the start. Find effective ways to share or get help from others.

If you find yourself in an angry conversation with the person in your care **in your head, get it out in the open.**

- Find a counselor or therapist to talk to.

- Talk to a neutral third party, even if it's by phone or e-mail.

- Tap into a local or online support group.

- Keep a journal.

Respite Time

Every caregiver needs respite time if she is to last. It may be hard to think of yourself and your needs at this time, but if you don't, your life will be consumed by your duties and you will burn out. Respite (a temporary break from responsibility) is not a luxury, it is a necessity.

Your care receiver's level of disability determines whether he or she can be left alone and for how long. Care options include—

- asking a family member or friend to stay with your survivor for an hour or two

- taking him or her to adult daycare (if ambulatory)

- employing a professional sitter or health care aide for a few hours a week or month

- hiring a college student (if skilled care is not needed) to stay with your care receiver

- enrolling the person in your care in a support group

Check with your local Area Agency on Aging for respite-care programs in your area. Larger churches often have outreach programs that include respite care.

However you are able to arrange for some help—and it will take some effort on your part, it won't happen by itself—commit to taking some time at least once a week to do something for yourself.

NOTE To make this happen you will have to defend this time because other things will demand to be made a priority. If you do not defend your respite time, you will not get it or the renewal it generates. Remember, caregiving is a marathon, not a sprint—respite time helps you finish the race.

Respite Zone

A respite zone is an area within your home set aside just for you, the caregiver. The idea is that this is your space. It can be your bedroom, the spare room, an office, or even a bench outside in the garden or on a porch. This is a place for you to take a break while the person in your care rests or is taken care of by someone else.

In creating your respite zone,

- Keep in mind what you want to do there. Reading? Painting? Writing? Gardening? Bubble bath?

- Identify the time you will use it—during nap time, when someone spells you? If you can only get a break at night after the person in your care is in bed, gardening probably won't do.

- Identify free space in your home—porches are good candidates, a spare room is perfect, maybe a corner of your bedroom. A screen can give you privacy if you can't close the door.

- Modify the space according to your needs—a reading chair with a lamp or a stereo headset. Keep whatever is necessary for your respite activity.

Your respite zone should be your creation alone. The goal is to give you a place of your own where you can find enjoyment in your own home and life. If searching the Internet is fun for you, your zone will be different from someone who wants to take a bubble bath and listen to soft music. Creative projects such as painting, sewing, writing, baking, gardening, and photography are excellent ways to absorb your attention and take your mind off your responsibilities.

Your respite zone should be just for you. You need to feel secure that your things are safe and will not be disturbed or discarded. It is important for your care receiver to understand that this space is yours.

Tip

It is not selfish to set aside space and time for yourself, because if you fail to give yourself space, time, and the opportunity to be with your own thoughts, your caregiving journey will be harder on you than it has to be.

Taking care of a debilitated (weakened) family member or friend who may not recover completely can be an all-consuming job. However, if you allow it to consume all of you because you do not demand some time and space for yourself, what will happen to the person in your care when you collapse?

Respite care is not a luxury. It is necessary for the well-being of the person in your care and for you.

Changes in Attitude Relieve Stress

Here are some suggestions to help reduce your stress level:

- Learn to say no. Good boundaries improve relationships.

- Control your attitude: Don't dwell on what you lack or what you can't change.

- Appreciate what you have and can do.

- Find simple ways to have fun: Play a board game, organize family photos, listen to music you enjoy, read the biography of an inspiring person.

- Learn a time-management tool, like making a to-do list (specifically include items that you enjoy).

- Knowledge is empowering; get information about the person's condition.

- Limit coffee and caffeine.

- Find a support system and nurture it.

- Share your feelings with someone who wants to listen.

- Keep a gratitude journal—record three new things you are grateful for every day.

- Memorize an inspiring poem.

> **NOTE** The #1 thing you can do to improve your situation is to acknowledge your role. A survey of family caregivers by the National Family Caregivers Association showed that spouse caregivers often refuse to accept that caregiving is a separate role to the role of spouse. The survey found that shifting this attitude—accepting that caregiving is a separate role—had a profound impact on their situation.

The job of long-term caregiving is too big for one person—no matter how much love the caregiver has for the care receiver. Ask for and accept help from as many sources as you can find.

Outside Activities

Successful caregivers don't give up their own enjoyable activities. Many organizations have respite care programs to provide a break for caregivers. Other family members are often willing—even pleased—to spend time with the person. It may be possible to have respite care on a regular basis. Keep a list of the people you can ask for help once in a while.

If your friends want to know how they can help ease your burden, ask them to:

- telephone and be a good listener as you may voice strong feelings
- offer words of appreciation for your efforts
- share a meal
- help you find useful information about community resources
- show genuine interest
- stop by or send cards, letters, pictures, or humorous newspaper clippings

- share the workload

- help hire a relief caregiver

It helps to remember the saying, "Grant me the serenity to accept the things I cannot change, the courage to change the things I can, and the wisdom to know the difference."

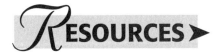

RESOURCES ➤

Caregiver Survival Resources
www.caregiver911.com
A comprehensive list linking caregiving information and services for general issues and specific chronic illnesses.

Caring.com
Help with concerns about caregiving and advice from trusted experts in medicine, legal matters, finances, housing, and family issues, as well as community support from caregivers like you.
www.caring.com

Center for Family Caregivers/Tad Publishing Co.
www.caregiving.com or www.familycaregivers.org
Develops and distributes educational materials on caregiving, including a newsletter. Caregiving informational kits are $5 each; please specify new, seasoned, and transitioning caregiver when requesting a kit.

Lotsa Helping Hands
www.lotsahelpinghands.com
Provides a free-of-charge Web service that allows family, friends, neighbors, and colleagues to assist more easily with daily meals, rides, shopping, baby-sitting, and errands that may become a burden during times of medical crisis.

My Calm Space

www.mycalmspace.com

A useful Web site with helpful ideas and techniques for finding wellness through meditation.

National Alliance for Caregiving

4720 Montgomery Lane, 5th Floor
Bethesda, MD 20184
www.caregiving.org

The Alliance is a non-profit coalition of national organizations focusing on issues of family caregiving.

National Family Caregivers Association

10400 Connecticut Avenue, Suite 500
Kensington, MD 20895
(800) 896-3650
info@thefamilycaregiver.org
www.thefamilycaregiver.org

Free member benefits include Take Care!, a quarterly newsletter.

Today's Caregiver Magazine

6365 Taft Street, Suite 3003
Hollywood, FL 33024
(800) 829-2734
www.caregiver.com/magazine

Bimonthly magazine dedicated to caregivers.

Well Spouse Association

63 West Main Street, Suite H
Freehold, NJ 07728
(800) 838-0879
info@wellspouse.org
www.wellspouse.org

Publishes Mainstay, a bimonthly newsletter and provides networking/local support groups.

Check with your local church or health facility to see if they sponsor **Share the Care** teams.

Publications

A Caregiver's Survival Guide: How to Stay Healthy When Your Loved One Is Sick, by Kay Marshall Strom. Intervarsity Press, 2000.

Care for the Family Caregiver: A Place to Start, a report prepared by HIP Health Plan of New York and National Alliance for Caregiving. Available at www.caregiving.org

Caring for Yourself While Caring for Others: A Caregiver's Survival and Renewal Guide, by Lawrence M. Brammer. Vantage Press, 1999.

Caring for Yourself While Caring for Your Aging Parents: How to Help, How to Survive, by Claire Berman. Henry Holt, 1996.

Helping Yourself Help Others: A Book for Caregivers, by Rosalynn Carter, with Susan Golant. Random House/Time Books, 1995.
(800) 733-3000
Plenty of basic information for caregivers.

A Family Caregiver Speaks Up: It Doesn't Have To Be this Hard, by Suzanne Geffen Mintz. Capital Books, 2007.

Mainstay: For the Well Spouse of the Chronically Ill, by Maggie Strong.

Positive Caregiver Attitudes by James Sherman, PhD.

The Emotional Survival Guide for Caregivers by Barry J. Jacobs, PsyD. The Guilford Press, 2006.

The Fearless Caregiver: How to Get the Best Care From Your Loved One and Still Have a Life of Your Own, by Gary Barg. Capital Books, 2001.

If you don't have home access to the Internet, ask your local library to help you locate any Web site.

Activities of Daily Living

Activities of Daily Living

Personal Hygiene

As a caregiver, you may find that some of your time each day will be devoted to assisting the person in your care with personal hygiene. This includes bathing, shampooing, oral or mouth care, shaving, and foot care.

The Basin Bath

If the person in your care can be in a chair or wheelchair, you can give a sponge bath at the sink.

1. Make sure the room is warm.

2. Gather supplies—disposable gloves, mild soap, washcloth, washbasin, lotion, comb, electric razor, shampoo—and clean clothes.

3. Use good body mechanics (position)—keep your feet separated, stand firmly, bend your knees, and keep your back in neutral.

4. Offer the urinal.

5. Wash the face first.

6. Wash the rest of the upper body.

7. If the person can stand, wash the genitals. If the person is too weak to stand, wash the lower part of the body in the bed.

 NOTE Make sure the person in your care uses his own razor, especially if he has hepatitis B or C.

The Tub Bath

If the person in your care has good mobility and is strong enough to get in and out of the tub, he or she may enjoy a tub bath. Be sure there are grab bars, a bath bench, and a rubber mat so the person doesn't slide. (It may be easier to sit at bench level rather than at the bottom of the tub.) Use the following steps:

1. Make sure the room is a comfortable temperature.

2. Gather supplies—disposable gloves for the caregiver, mild soap, washcloth, lotion, comb, electric razor, shampoo—and clean clothes.

3. Check the water temperature before the person gets in.

4. Guide the person into the tub. Have the person use the grab bars. (Don't let the person grab you and pull you down.)

5. Help the person wash.

6. Empty the tub and then help the person get out.

7. Guide the person to use the grab bars while getting out. OR you can have the person stand up and then sit on the bath bench. Swing first one leg, then the other leg, over the edge of the tub. Help him stand.

8. Put a towel on a chair or the toilet lid and have the person sit there to dry off.

9. Apply lotion to any skin that appears dry.

10. Help the person dress.

BATHING IN THE TUB

If a bath bench is not used, many people feel more secure if they turn on to their side and then get on their knees before rising from the tub. This is a very helpful way to get out of the tub if the person is unsteady.

The Shower

Before starting, be sure the shower floor is not slippery. Also make sure there are grab bars, a bath bench, and a rubber mat so the person doesn't slide. A removable shower head is also useful.

1. Make sure the room is a comfortable temperature.

2. Explain to the person what you are going to do.

3. Provide a shower stool in case he or she needs to sit.

4. Gather supplies—mild soap, washcloth, washbasin, comb, electric razor, shampoo—and clean clothes.

5. Turn on the cold water and then the hot to prevent burns. Test and adjust the water temperature before the person gets in. Use gentle water pressure.

6. First, spray and clean the less sensitive parts of the body such as the feet.

7. For safety, ask the person to hold the grab bar or to sit on the shower stool.

8. Move the water hose around the person rather than asking the person to move.

9. Assist in washing as needed.

10. Guide the person out of the shower and wrap with a towel. Turn the water off.

11. Apply lotion to skin that appears dry.

12. If necessary, have the person sit on a stool or on the toilet lid.

13. Assist in drying and dressing.

NOTE Remove from the bathing area all electrical equipment that could get wet.

Most patients with liver disease are not bedbound and therefore are able to participate in ADLs. If the person in your care needs bed bath or bed shampooing, please refer to *The Comfort of Home: A Complete Guide for Caregivers*, 3rd Edition.

Shampooing the Hair

Keeping the hair and scalp clean improves blood flow to the scalp and keeps the hair healthy. Women especially may consider it a special treat to have their hair styled. Shampooing can be done anytime the person in your care is not overly tired. Before a bath may be the most convenient time. Adopt a system that is easiest for you and the person in your care.

SHAMPOOING
To make washing easy, dilute the shampoo in a bottle before pouring it on the hair.

Never use an electric razor if the person is receiving oxygen. Make sure you wear gloves during shaving if the person in your care has hepatitis B or C.

Dressing

Dressing a person with disabilities can be made easier by following a routine. Before you begin, lay the clothes out in the order in which they will be put on.

- Dress the person while he or she is sitting.

- Use adaptive equipment like a button hook and shoehorn.

- Use loose clothes that are easy to put on and have elastic waistbands, Velcro® fasteners, and front openings.

- Use bras that open and close in front.

- Use tube socks.

- Dress the weaker side first.

- For a person who is confined to bed, use a gown that closes in the back. This will make it easier when using a bedpan or urinal.

Allow the person to choose their clothes if possible. This helps the patient have some control. They may have certain favorite clothes they may want to wear more often.

NOTE For a person who is confined to bed, be sure to smooth out all wrinkles in the clothes and bedding to prevent pressure sores.

Toileting

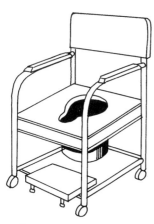

▲ *Portable commode chair*

Always wear disposable gloves when helping with toileting. This prevents the spread of disease. Wash your hands before and after providing care.

Using a Portable Commode

1. Gather the portable commode, toilet tissue, a basin, a cup of water, a washcloth or paper towel, soap, and a towel.

2. Wash your hands.

3. Help the person onto the commode.

4. Offer toilet tissue when the person is finished.

5. Pour a cup of warm water on female genitalia.

6. Pat the area dry with a paper towel.

7. Offer a washcloth so the person can wash his or her hands.

8. Remove the pail from under the seat, empty it, rinse it with clear water, and empty the water into the toilet.

9. Wash your hands.

TOILET SAFETY
Use Velcro® with tape on the back and attach it to the back of the toilet or commode seat to keep the lid from falling.

Using the Bathroom Toilet

If the mobile person is missing the toilet, get a toilet seat in a color that is different from the floor color. This may help him see the toilet better. If he is failing to cleanse the anal area or failing to wash his hands, use tact to encourage him to do so. This will help prevent the spread of infections.

Incontinence

Incontinence is the leakage of urine or a bowel movement over which the person has no control. In addition to bladder management medications, treatments can include bladder training, exercises to strengthen the pelvic floor (Kegel exercises), biofeedback, surgery, electrical muscle stimulator, urinary catheter, prosthetic devices, or external collection devices. Talk to the doctor about the options or treatments for the person in your care.

Optimal Bowel Function

Maintaining good bowel function can be a challenge, especially in individuals who are unable to get out of bed and get little exercise.

People with liver disease may need to take certain medicines that increase the frequency of urination and bowel movements. Therefore, it is important to make sure toilet facilities are readily available and easy to reach.

- Bowel movement is an important issue for the care receiver with end-stage liver disease. People with end-stage liver disease should have 3–4 formed (pudding-like) bowel movements per day to decrease risk of confusion.

- Serve fruits, vegetables, and bran.

- Be sure the person in your care drinks 2 quarts (8 glasses) of water daily (or an amount directed by the doctor).

- Provide a chance for daily exercise.

Diarrhea

Diarrhea (loose, watery stools) occurs when the intestines push stool along before the water in them can be reabsorbed (taken up) by the body. This condition can be caused by viral stomach flu, antibiotics, or other medications, or stress anxiety. Remember that it might be too much lactulose when end-stage liver patients develop diarrhea.

Diarrhea in people who are immobile is often caused by impaction. This is a blockage formed by hardened stool, with liquid stool passing around it. This must always be taken into consideration, because the usual treatments for diarrhea would be extremely dangerous if the diarrhea is being caused by impaction.

Tip First line of care in people with end-stage liver disease and diarrhea is always to decrease the lactulose dose. Do **not** use antidiarrheal medication. Instead call the person in your care's liver doctor for further instructions.

Hemorrhoids

Hemorrhoids are swollen inflamed veins around the anus. They cause tenderness, pain, and bleeding. Hemorrhoids are a common problem in people with end-stage liver disease. To treat hemorrhoids, you should do the following:

- Be sure to keep anal area clean with premoistened tissues.

- Apply zinc oxide or petroleum jelly to the area.

- Relieve itching by using cold compresses on the anus for 10 minutes several times a day.

- Ask the doctor about suppositories.

Call the Doctor

- if blood from the hemorrhoids is dark red or brown and heavy

- if bleeding continues for more than one week

- if bleeding seems to occur for no reason

- if the stool seems black

Control of Infection in the Home

Common health practices such as frequent hand-washing are necessary to avoid the risk of bacterial, viral, and fungal infections.

 To minimize the chance of infection
- Always start with the cleanest area and work toward the dirtiest area.
- Always wash your hands before and after contact with the person in your care and with other people.
- Always wear disposable gloves when giving personal care.
- Always wash hands well when returning from a trip outside the house.
- Always wash your hands after using the toilet.

Cleaning Techniques

The following techniques will help cut the chance of infection in the home.

Caregiver Handwashing

- Hand-washing is the single most effective way to prevent the spread of infection or germs.

- Use bottle-dispensed hand soap.

- If the person in your care has an infection, use antimicrobial soap.

- Rub your hands for at least 30 seconds to produce lots of lather. Do this away from running water so that the lather is not washed away.

- Use a nailbrush on your nails; keep nails trimmed.

- Wash front and back of hands, between fingers, and at least 2 inches up your wrists.

- Repeat the process.

- Dry your hands on a clean towel or a paper towel.

Handling Soiled Laundry

- Do not carry soiled linen close to your body.

- Never shake dirty items or put soiled linens on the floor. They can contaminate (infect) the floor and germs will be spread throughout the house on the soles of shoes.

- Store infected soiled linen in a leak-proof plastic bag and tie it closed.

- Bag soiled laundry in the same place it is used.

- Wash soiled linen separately from other clothes.

- Fill the machine with hot water, add bleach (no more than 1/4 cup) and detergent. Rinse twice and then dry.

- Clean the washer by running it through a cycle with 1 cup of bleach or other disinfectant to kill germs.

- Use rubber gloves when handling soiled laundry.

- Wash your hands.

Be extra careful if blood is present

NOTE If urine is highly concentrated due to a bladder infection or dehydration, do not use bleach. The combination of ammonia in the urine and bleach can cause toxic fumes.

Disposal of Body Fluids

- Wear disposable gloves (recommended for handling all body fluids).

- Flush liquid and solid waste down the toilet.

- Place used dressings and disposable (throwaway) pads in a sturdy plastic bag, tie securely, and place in a sealed container for collection.

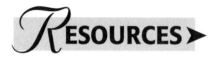

RESOURCES ➤

Meeting Life's Challenges
9042 Aspen Grove Lane
Madison, WI 53717
Fax (608) 824-0403
www.meetinglifeschallenges.com
E-mail: help@meetinglifeschallenges.com
Offers a guide called Dressing Tips and Clothing Resources for Making Life Easier, by Shelley P. Schwarz, a guide to dressing for people with disabilities plus more than 100 resources for custom clothing.

National Association for Continence (NAFC)
P.O. Box 8310
Spartanburg, SC 29305-8310
(800) 252-3337; (864) 579-7900; Fax (864) 579-7902
www.nafc.org
NAFC is a leading source of education and support to the public about the diagnosis, treatments, and management alternatives for incontinence.

If you don't have home access to the Internet, ask your local library to help you locate any Web site.

Therapies

Therapies

*T*he following information is provided for your general knowledge. It IS NOT a substitute for training with professional therapists.

Physical Therapy

Physical therapy is part of the process of relearning how to function after an injury, illness, or period of inactivity. If muscles are not used, they shorten and tighten, making joint motion painful.

What a Physical Therapist Does

A physical therapist treats a person to relieve pain, build up and restore muscle function, and maintain the best possible performance. The therapist does this by using physical means such as active and passive exercise, massage, heat, water, and electricity. Broadly speaking, a physical therapist:

- sets up the goals of treatment with patient and family

- shows how to use special equipment

- instructs in routine daily functions

- teaches safe ways to move

- sets up and teaches an exercise program

The American Physical Therapy Association, often located in the state capital, can provide a list of licensed therapists.

What a Physical Therapist Determines

Depending on a person's physical condition, a therapist may work on range-of-motion exercises, correct body positions when resting, devices to help the person in your care, and other simple ways to improve daily functions.

A physical therapist checks things that can affect a person's daily activities—

- the person's attitude toward his situation

- how well he can move his muscles and joints (range of motion)

- his ability to see, smell, hear, and feel

- what he can do on his own and what he needs to learn

- his equipment needs, now and in the future

- what can be improved in the home to make moving around safer and more comfortable

- who can and will help to give support

Range-of-Motion (ROM) Exercises

The purpose of range-of-motion exercises is to relieve pain, maintain normal body alignment (positions), help prevent skin swelling and breakdown, and promote bone formation. A ROM exercise program should be started before deformities develop. Here are some things to do when you are asked to help with exercises at home:

- Communicate what you are doing.

- Use the flats of both hands, not the fingertips, to hold a body part.

Joints Used in ROM

▲ shoulder

▲ hip

▲ shoulders

▲ finger/thumb

▲ feet, ankle, toe

▲ hands

▲ wrists

▲ elbows

▲ neck

- Take each movement only as far as the joint will go into a comfortable stretch. (Mild discomfort is okay, but it should go away quickly.)

- Do each exercise 3 to 5 times.

- Use slow steady movements to help relax muscles and increase joint range.

- If joints are swollen and painful, exercise very gently.

Massage Therapy

Massage therapy increases circulation (blood flow), reduces muscle tension, and helps a person relax. It can be very useful to people who experience problems with rigidity (stiffness). Massage should be part of an overall fitness program that includes regular movement and exercise.

Select a massage therapist who is certified by the American Massage Therapy Association. Talk to the therapist about methods. The care receiver should provide feedback during the massage in the event of any discomfort. Self-massage and massage provided by the caregiver are also possible. Using items such as wooden rollers or hand-held electric massagers will allow you or the person in your care to apply gentle pressure to tight areas of the body. These items can be purchased at most drug or department stores. Massage services are often not covered by health insurance.

Pet Therapy

A cat, bird, or dog can bring great joy to people. Having animals in the home improves the mental and emotional health of their owners. It also provides movement and exercise.

Animals also lessen the boredom and fear caused by loneliness. According to research, pets can—

• lower blood pressure and heart rate

• improve mobility and flexibility (through stroking, grooming, and walking the pet)

• satisfy the human need for touch and caring for another

Before selecting a dog, check canine-assistant programs in your area. Dogs that were rejected from the program may be ideal for the person in your care.

• Choose a mature dog that is housetrained; do not get a puppy.

• Have a dog or cat neutered or spayed to lessen the chance of roaming.

• Keep up all pet vaccinations.

• Never clean pet cages or feeding dishes in the kitchen sink.

 Be aware that animals carry bacteria and intestinal parasites. Individuals with weakened immune systems should not change the litter box or pick up outside waste and should wash their hands frequently.

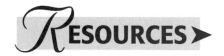

RESOURCES ➤

Canine Companions for Independence
(800) 572-BARK (1-800-572-2275).
www.caninecompanions.org
A national nonprofit organization that enhances the lives of children and adults with disabilities by providing highly-trained assistance dogs and ongoing support to ensure quality partnerships.

Delta Society
875 124th Ave NE, Suite 101
Bellevue, WA 98005
(425) 226-7357; Fax (425) 235-1076
www.deltasociety.org
E-Mail: info@deltasociety.org
Provides information on the human-animal bond and information on how to obtain a service animal.

National Center of Complementary and Alternative Medicine Clearinghouse
(888) 644-6226
www.nccam.nih.gov

Contact your local **Humane Society** for information about pet therapy.

If you don't have home access to the Internet, ask your local library to help you locate any Website.

Special Challenges

Special Challenges

Communication

Communication is the ability to speak, understand speech, read, write, and gesture. Nonverbal messages are given through silence, body movements, or facial expression. Be aware that words can carry one message, the body another.

People with liver failure can experience a condition called hepatic encephalopathy. The symptoms can range from forgetfulness and confusion to coma. This is a result of ammonia building up in the body. The damaged liver is not able to get rid of ammonia effectively, resulting in accumulation. People with hepatic encephalopathy become confused, slow to respond, move slowly, have shaking hands, and are not able to understand things as they did before (decreased understanding, comprehension) etc.

- The communication problem may involve talking or understanding.

- The person may be able to say words at one time and then not at another, or may repeat the same word over and over.

To communicate better with the person in your care, try:

- getting the person's attention by lightly touching her arm before speaking

- speaking slowly and simply

- asking questions that require simple yes/no answers

- providing opportunities for the person to hear speech

- helping the person communicate frustrations

- pacing activities, because the person will tire easily

Sexual Expression

A disability does not equate with loss of sexuality. The needs for intimacy and sharing do not change, although the ability to move in the usual manner may have changed. To improve your spouse's ability to exercise sexual expression, try to increase his or her self-esteem and downplay the role of "patient." Ask your health care professional about assistive devices and techniques for enhanced sexual activities.

It is important that the caregiver and the care receiver understand that liver disease can result in certain chemical changes in the body that change sexuality. It is important to talk about this and seek medical help when appropriate.

When people have cirrhosis, estrogen (a female hormone) is not removed properly, resulting in its accumulation in the body. This can be problematic for men as this can result in enlarged breasts (gynecomastia) and increased emotions (e.g., they cry more). This also changes the estrogen/testosterone balance and can result in change in libido and erectile dysfunction. These problems can have a significant impact on sexuality. It is important to recognize and discuss with the care receiver's sexual partner. Also, discuss with the doctor. In some cases, testosterone injections may help.

Tip

It is important to bring up any issue regarding sexuality during the person in your care's doctor's visit. Medical professionals often overlook these problems and do not ask caregivers about them. However, fixing this problem plays an important role in improving quality of life.

Depression

People with liver disease may have worsening negative emotions and mental attitudes. This is especially true when future events regarding liver transplant and how long the wait will be are not predictable. Personality changes with chronic illness can be dramatic, and people with worsening conditions can suffer personality changes that are as permanent as the disease. People with liver disease may feel guilty if the disease is a result of their life style/behavior.

Common Fears of a Person with a Chronic Illness

- loss of self-image

- loss of control over life

- loss of independence and fear of abandonment

- fear of living alone and being lonely

- fear of death

You can help deal with these powerful emotions by:

- pointing out the person's strengths and focusing on small successes

- restoring areas of control to the person by giving as many choices as possible

- finding new ways for the person to adjust to limitations

- providing insight into sources of meaning in life

- changing your attitude about the person's disability

- recognizing that humor is healing and providing large doses of laughter to stimulate a positive attitude, providing humorous books, comics, cartoons, television, or movies

- allowing the person to cry at hearing news of a diagnosis

- allowing for the power of silence

- providing opportunities for peer support and friendship (which works exceptionally well with the elderly)

Certain medicines used in patients with liver disease can increase depression.

Dealing with Boredom

Boredom is another problem for people who are ill, and fighting it can take all your creativity. Try—

- watching funny movies

- taking car or bus trips depending on the care receiver's condition

- listening to music, especially from the person's youth

- taking up hobbies

- going to social events

- playing board games and card games

- attending public library discussion clubs and using large-print or talking books

- joining activist organizations like the League of Women Voters and Gray Panthers

- spending time with others in similar difficulties—in religious groups, recreation centers, AA or NA meetings, or the YMCA/YWCA

- being involved in volunteer service organizations such as the Retired & Senior Volunteer Program

- using a computer and accessing sites on the Internet (which helps prevent loneliness through interesting activity and provides the ability to communicate with family and friends through e-mail)

> **Tip**
> A computer is ideal for the person who has difficulty writing, which can happen as a result of hepatic encephalopathy, and it can make life simpler and more enjoyable for anyone.

Pain Management

Pain is not a common problem with liver disease. Some people may experience mild pain/discomfort in some cases. Ascites—water in the abdomen—can cause pain or discomfort. Usually, pain is a sign of something seriously wrong and medical attention is necessary.

If the person in your care is experiencing chronic pain, please refer to *The Comfort of Home: A Complete Guide for Caregivers* (3rd edition) for help in pain management.

Abuse

Abusive behavior is never acceptable. Though tensions can mount in the most loving families and result in frustration and anger, an emotionally damaging or physically forceful response is not okay. When this happens, call for a time-out, and call for help.

Physical abuse usually begins in the process of giving or receiving personal help. For instance, the caregiver might be too rough during dressing or grooming, or the care receiver might accidentally scratch the caregiver during a transfer. Once anger and frustration reach this level, abuse by either person may become frequent.

The dangers of physical abuse are easy to see, but emotional abuse is also unhealthy and damaging. Continued shaming, harsh criticism, or controlling behaviors can damage the self-esteem of either person.

Dealing With Anger and Abuse

Communicating When the Person in Your Care Is Angry

To help diffuse a situation so that it doesn't become a problem, here is how to communicate with someone who is angry.

DO

- Be patient, calm, courteous, sympathetic, and show your concern and caring.

- Be open to listening to the person explain the problem before you respond with an answer.

- Look at the problem from the point of view of the person in your care.

- Remember, the person is upset about a situation, not you.

DON'T

- Be defensive and angry.

- Raise your voice (yelling never helps).

- Intimidate the person in your care.

It is important that you, as caregiver, manage your anger. Ask, "What can we do to make things better?" Think about your own feelings and what button is being pushed. Understanding what is upsetting you will help you from losing control.

Tips You Can Use to Diffuse Anger

1. Communicate. Tell the person in your care that you understand or are trying to. "If it happened to me, I'd be angry too."

2. Remind the person that she has choices. Because of her anger she may not realize the choices she has.

3. Affirm her feelings. Say, "I see you are angry."

4. Repeat yourself like a broken record. Softly repeat what is necessary.

What You Can Do

Help the person in your care identify a trusted person who can be called on for help. The Adult Protective Services Agency—a component of the human service agency in most states—is typically responsible for investigating reports of domestic elder abuse and providing families with help and guidance. Other professionals who may be able to help include doctors or nurses, police officers, lawyers, and social workers.

Transportation and Travel

Transportation

Ask your specialist if the person is able to travel out of state, or out of the country.

There is a network of transportation services, public and private, that will pick up the disabled and the elderly at their homes. These services rely on vans and paid drivers and run on a schedule to specific locations. Free transportation is available from community volunteer organizations, although most public services charge on a sliding scale.

Many states ensure transportation to necessary medical care for Medicaid recipients. Check with your local Medicaid office to see if you qualify.

Community transportation services are provided by:

- home health care agencies
- public health departments
- religious organizations
- civic clubs
- the local American Red Cross
- the Area Agency on Aging
- local public transportation companies

Travel

Some group tours and cruise lines cater to the elderly or disabled traveler. Before traveling long distances with a person who has a chronic condition, however, consult the person's doctor.

 TRAVEL PLANNING
If you, as the primary caregiver, are traveling for an extended period, consider investing in a long-distance pager with a toll-free pager number so you can be reached in case of emergency.

Checklist Travel for the Person with a Chronic Condition

✓ Let the person's primary care doctor know of your travel plans.

✓ Take more of the person's medications than needed, along with a list of names and dosages. Make sure to include brand names and generic names. Names of most medicines are often different in other countries.

✓ Check with the doctor to see what immunization is recommended if traveling to high-risk areas.

✓ Take a list of all medical conditions.

✓ Use a Medic-Alert identification bracelet for the person in care.

✓ Take a copy of his EKG.

✓ Read his insurance policy before taking the trip to see how "emergency" is defined.

✓ If medical care is needed during the trip, get copies of all bills to support claims for reimbursement.

✓ Check into reciprocal agreements between the person's health plan and a provider in the area you will visit.

✓ If you anticipate the need for medical care, call ahead or ask your HMO to help you make doctor's appointments in the new location.

✓ Consider buying traveler's insurance. Study the policy terms regarding pre-existing conditions. READ THE FINE PRINT.

✓ Check that medical equipment is insured for loss or theft.

✓ Consider taking a portable grab bar on the trip.

✓ If traveling to a foreign country, see if the policy allows for medical evacuation.

✓ Take the person's health insurance card and the HMO's toll free number for travelers.

✓ Take copies of the pages in the insurance benefits booklet dealing with emergency access.

✓ Carry a card listing phone numbers of next-of-kin in case of illness during the trip.

✓ Carry a copy of the Consular Information Sheet of the country you are visiting.

✓ Write the primary care doctor's number and beeper number on the health insurance card, along with the date of the last tetanus injection.

✓ If taking a cruise, ask if a doctor with experience in emergency medicine or family practice will be on board.

✓ Keep a copy of the original prescription if traveling with medicines. May need a note from the doctor if traveling with syringes and needles.

✓ Tell the travel agent or airline that you will require a wheelchair and ask to have your request noted on the ticket.

✓ Call ahead to the airport, bus station or train station to request assistance.

✓ If a flight is delayed for more than four hours, an airline has a duty to provide a meal that is comparable to the meal offered on the flight—if asked for by the passenger.

Travel Emergencies

In the event of an emergency abroad, contact American Citizen Services (ACS) in the foreign offices of American consulates and embassies.

American Citizens Services will assist with:

- lists of doctors, dentists, hospitals, and clinics

- informing the family if an American becomes ill or injured while traveling

- helping arrange transportation to the United States on a commercial flight (must be paid by the traveler)

- explaining various options and costs for return of remains or burial

- helping locate you, the caregiver, if you are traveling when a family member becomes ill

Travel and Living Wills

If a person becomes disabled with a life-threatening illness while traveling, the medical personnel in foreign countries may not accept the validity of an advance directive (or any other form a personal attorney has drawn up). If a person is traveling and has an illness that requires breathing devices or other life-prolonging treatments, it may be impossible to end the treatment without a medical evacuation back to the United States. However, there a few basic precautions you can take to ensure that a person's wishes are carried out:

- Take a copy of the living will on the trip. Let any other traveling companions know where it is packed.

- Take health-care directive documents with you.

- If traveling in the United States, consider signing the form used in the state where you might be traveling.

TRAVELING ABROAD

When traveling in tropical countries, use the standard traveler's rule: boil it, peel it, cook it, or forget it!

Traveling with Medications

Traveling with medications should not stop you and your care receiver from enjoying travel in the United States and abroad. Some tours or cruise lines require a note from the doctor stating that the person is fit to travel. Here are some tips when traveling with medications:

- Bring enough medication to last through your trip plus some extras.

- Pack your meds in a carry-on bag—luggage can stray or become lost.

- Keep all medication in original containers with original prescription labels.

- Make a list of the medications the person takes, and why, with brand and generic names. Make a copy and pack one copy separately.

- Make arrangements for refrigerating the medication if needed.

- If intravenous medication is used, carry a used-needle container. Get a note from the doctor specifically allowing you to travel with syringes and bottles in your carry-on luggage if traveling by plane.

- Bring the person insurance ID card, plus instructions for accessing a physician where you are going.

- Bring the doctor name and contact information, in case of emergency.

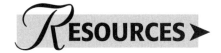

RESOURCES

Abuse

National Center for Elder Abuse (NCEA)
1201 15th Street, NW
Suite 350
Washington, DC 20005-2842
(202) 898-2586
Fax (202) 898-2583
www.elderabusecenter.org
Offers fact sheets, reporting numbers, news, publications, and resources.

AIDS Resources

CDC National Prevention Information Network
P.O. Box 6003
Rockville, MD 20849-6003
(800) 458-5231
Fax (301) 562-1001 or (888) 282-7681
www.cdcnpin.org
Offers free government publications and information about resources on HIV/AIDS, STDs, and tuberculosis.

National AIDS HOTLINE
(800) 342-AIDS (2437)
(800) 344-SIDA (Spanish) 8 a.m.–2 a.m. EST 7 days per week
(800) AIDS-889 (TTY) 10 a.m.–10 p.m. EST Monday through Friday
Operates 24 hours a day, 7 days a week and offers general information and local referrals to support groups for caregivers.

National Institute on Aging
NIA Information Center
P.O. Box 8057
Gaithersburg, MD 20898-8057
(800) 222-2225
(800) 222-4225 (TTY)
Fax (301) 589-3014
www.nih.gov/nia
A government program that provides free publications on aging and related health issues.

Senior Action in a Gay Environment (SAGE)
305 7th Avenue 16th Floor
New York, NY 10001
(212) 741-2247
www.sageusa.org
Provides HIV/AIDS information and referrals for people age 50 and older.

Social Security Administration
(800) SSA-1213 (800) 772-1213
www.ssa.gov

OR

Contact your local SS office.
Has two disability benefit programs that provide financial assistance to eligible AIDS patients.

National Organization for Victim Assistance (NOVA)
1730 Park Road, NW
Washington, D.C. 20010
(800) 879-6682 (TRY-NOVA) 24-hour hotline
www.try-nova.org
A nonprofit organization that provides the name and number of a victim's assistance support group in your area, and free informational brochures. They also provide training in crisis response.

Centers for Disease Control and Prevention
(877) FYI-TRIP (394-8747)
Fax requests: (888) 232-3299
www.cdc.gov
Provides recommendations on vaccinations and health data for travel to specific countries; also provides information about diseases such as malaria and yellow fever.

Consular Information Program
Bureau of Consular Affairs
State Department
(202) 647-3000 for automatic fax
(202) 647-5225 for recorded messages
www.travel.state.gov
Provides travel advisory information and emergency assistance. Ask for a complete set of Department of State, Bureau of Consular Affairs publications including "Medical Information for Americans Traveling Abroad."

Travel Assistance International
9200 Keystone Crossing Suite 300
Indianapolis, IN 46240
(800) 821-2828
(317) 575-2652
Fax (317)-575-2659
www.travelassistance.com
A for-profit company which provides members with worldwide, 24-hours-per-day comprehensive travel services such as on-site emergency medical payments, emergency medical transportation, and assistance with medication replacement.

If you don't have home access to the Internet, ask your local library to help you locate any Web site.

Diet, Nutrition, and Exercise

Diet, Nutrition, and Exercise

A person's quality of life can often be improved by focusing on those aspects of health that can be changed. Good health has a lot to do with what you do each and every day. Eating right and being physically active are areas in which you can be in control. The lifestyle habits you choose can have a lot to do with feeling good today and staying healthy tomorrow.

Proper nutrition is basic to good health. An older person's diet should avoid high-calorie, low-nutrient food. As the body ages, a person has to make more of an effort to eat wisely. However, there is no need to change food habits to drastically lower fat intake.

General Nutritional Guidelines for the Person with Advanced Liver Disease

Here is a brief summary of nutrition suggestions for the person in your care.

People with liver disease should eat normally, following a well-balanced diet complete with chicken, fish, vegetables, and fruits. The person in your care should avoid salt as much as possible. The maximum daily allowance is 2000 mg/day.

He should also avoid anything out of a can, as well as frozen or preserved foods. These types of foods are usually full of salt. Restaurant food is also high in salt. Fresh home-cooked food is best. Avoid excess vitamin A and iron supplements. Whatever is in the food naturally is ok. Make sure the person in your care avoids alcohol.

A person with liver disease should not eat raw shellfish. Be sure that he drinks 5 to 6 glasses of water daily (check with your doctor). The person with liver disease should limit caffeine intake to 1 to 2 cups/day. He should not eat large quantities of red meat. Make sure the person in your care takes a calcium supplements to avoid bone thinning.

 Use every means possible to perk up the appetite. Make sure the person's dentures fit correctly and that his or her glasses are adequate. We eat with our eyes before we ever touch our food.

Boosting Calorie or Protein Intake

If the person in your care has muscle wasting, which can happen with advanced liver disease, you may want to increase calorie and protein intake.

- Offer most of the food when the person is most hungry.

- Encourage the person to eat food with the fingers if it increases intake.

- Add non-fat powdered milk to any food with liquid in it, such as desserts, soups, gravy, and cereal.

- Add cottage cheese or ricotta cheese to casseroles, scrambled eggs, and desserts.

- Grate hard cheeses on bread, meats, vegetables, eggs, and casseroles.

- Add nuts, seeds, and wheat germ to breads, cereal, casseroles, and desserts.

- Offer 4–6 small meals throughout the day rather than 3 big meals a day.

Quick and Easy Snacks

- chocolate milk

- fruits, especially ripe bananas

- granola cookies

- hard-boiled eggs

- puddings

- raisins, nuts, prunes

- cottage cheese with fruits

Therapeutic Diets

Keep the doctor informed about the diet you follow. A special diet may be prescribed to:

- improve or maintain a person's health

- change the amount of bulk, as in a high fiber diet

- change the consistency of food, as in a special soft diet

- eliminate or decrease certain foods

- change the number of calories

Dehydration Prevention

People with liver disease often need to take water pills (diuretics). This can lead to some dehydration. Lactulose can result in diarrhea, which can also lead to dehydration. Therefore, it is important that you pay special attention to her hydration (amount of water she drinks).

It is important to remember that salt restriction is necessary to get rid of swelling: NOT *WATER RESTRICTION!*

People with liver disease can drink an average amount of water.

Avoid caffeinated beverages or limit them to 1–2 cups per day.

As a person ages, he feels less thirsty, so a special effort should be made to provide enough fluids. A person's fluid balance can be affected by medication, emotional stress, exercise, nourishment, general health, and the weather. Dehydration, especially in the elderly, can increase confusion and muscle weakness and cause nausea. Nausea, in turn, will prevent the person from wanting to eat, thereby causing more dehydration.

Preventative measures include:

- encouraging 6 cups of liquid every day (or an amount determined by the doctor)

- serving beverages at room temperature

- providing foods high in liquid (for example, watermelon)

- avoiding caffeine, which causes frequent urination and dehydration

Osteoporosis Prevention

Older people—especially women—suffer from osteoporosis, a condition that occurs when minerals are lost from the bones, thereby weakening them to the point where they break easily and are slow to heal. Patients with PBC (primary biliary cirrhosis) also have osteoporosis.

Osteoporosis can be prevented by:

- getting adequate vitamin D from sunshine a few times per week, and from fortified milk, fatty fish, or a vitamin supplement

- getting calcium from dairy foods; leafy vegetables such as kale and collards; broccoli; salmon; and sardines

 The National Institutes of Health recommends that postmenopausal women consume 1,500 milligrams of calcium daily to slow bone loss.

Recommended Daily Allowances for a Person Over Age 51

If you are concerned that an elderly person is malnourished, do a calorie check periodically. Recommended daily allowances are:

- women—1900 calories per day (63 grams fat)

- men—2200 calories per day (73 grams fat)

Checklist **Nutrition Assessment**

To assess nutrition risk for the person in your care, check the following questions. If the answer to most of the points is Yes, the person is at risk and you need to contact the doctor for a diet. Answer the questions every six months or whenever you notice big changes in weight or eating habits.

✓ Has she recently lost weight? About how much? _____ lbs.

✓ If the person with liver disease gains weight, be careful, it could be a sign of water retention. Please pay special attention to that.

✓ Has she had any recent appetite loss? _____ For how long? _____ (days, weeks, months)

✓ Does she have difficulty chewing? _____

✓ Does she have difficulty swallowing? _____

✓ Food allergies? _____

✓ Have you been given instructions about her diet? _____

✓ Does she eat fewer than 2 meals per day? _____

✓ Does she eat few fruits, vegetables, and dairy products? _____

✓ How many servings per day? Fruits _____ Vegetables _____ Dairy _____

✓ Does she drink more than 3 alcoholic beverages per day? _____

✓ Does she eat most of her meals alone? _____

✓ A special diet? _____

Weight Loss

This is not a diet book, but if you or your care receiver are overweight, then losing weight will require some change in diet. Whatever diet your doctor recommends, losing weight is a matter of taking in fewer calories than your body burns. It's like balancing a caloric checkbook, where calories are cash and weight is savings.

More calories burned than eaten = decreasing weight

More calories eaten than burned = increasing weight

 If you eat 10 calories more than you burn every day for a year, you'll gain 1 lb—3,600 calories = 1 lb.

If you do that for 20 years—just 10 calories more a day—at the end of 20 years, you'll have gained 20 lbs.

Ten calories is an insignificant amount of food. For many people, the overage is more in the hundreds-of-calories range. This simple equation may explain why 60 percent of Americans are either overweight or obese.

Diet and Nutrition Education

If you need reliable, well-organized, user-friendly advice about a healthy diet, get a copy of The No-Fad Diet from the American Heart Association (AHA). It is the only diet book the AHA has ever written, and it contains all the information you need about diet, exercise, and behavior change. It also contains sample meal plans, easy-to-prepare recipes, and information on starting an exercise program. One of the key features of the book is that it addresses the psychological component of changing behavior. The book is available at the American Stroke Association Web site, through online booksellers, or your local bookstore. In addition, AHA offers many cookbooks, all designed to combat cardiovascular disease and stroke.

A Foundation of Good Nutrition

Bringing good nutrition to the table takes planning, attention, and some imagination. A foundation to healthy eating can be found in the U.S. Department of Agriculture's **MyPyramid.** Making smart choices from each part of the pyramid is the best way to ensure one's body gets the balanced nutrition it needs. Here are some easy tips to make the most of every food group, and get the most from the calories eaten:

- **Focus on fruits.** Select fresh, frozen, canned, or dried over juices for most of your fruit choices.

- **Vary your vegetables.** Choose from a rainbow of colors—dark green, such as broccoli, kale, and spinach; orange, such as carrots, pumpkin, and sweet potatoes; yellow, such as yellow peppers and butternut squash.

- **Make half your grains whole.** When selecting cereals, breads, crackers, or pastas, look to see that the grains listed on the ingredient list are "whole." Whole grains provide a great source of fiber and can help in managing weight and controlling constipation.

- **Keep it lean.** Choose lean meats, fish, and poultry and bake, broil, or grill whenever possible. Try to vary your protein choices and add or substitute beans, peas, lentils, nuts, and seeds to what you eat.

- **Calcium counts.** Include 3 cups of low-fat or fat-free milk, yogurt, or equivalent of low-fat cheeses every day to maintain good bone health. Calcium-fortified foods and beverages can help fill the gap if you don't or can't consume milk.

- **Limit your fat, sugar, and salt.** These "extras" can add up! Check out the nutrition label on foods and look for foods low in saturated and trans fats. Sugars often only provide added calories with little added nutritional value. Choose and prepare foods with no salt.

Meeting the Challenges of Changing a Diet

If the person with liver disease is overweight, it is important that she lose weight slowly. This will help with better recovery after liver transplant. It will also help improve her overall health, especially if she has diabetes, high blood pressure, high cholesterol, back pain, hip or knee pain. Here are some simple steps to take to lose weight.

Good nutrition is the goal, but food is not just about nutrition. It is about emotions, culture, and being social. What and how we eat is so personal that changing eating habits can be difficult. Special diets and drastic fitness programs sometimes promise the quick fix, or even the cure. Yet, the best advice for care receivers is the same as for everyone: Eat a low-fat diet with a variety of grains, vegetables, and fruits, along with some high-protein foods like meat or dairy products; and balance how many calories you take in with physical activity.

Deciding to change is the first step. But the changes don't have to take place overnight. Start with the easy ones. Then, one by one, add more kinds of vegetables, reduce portion sizes, start eating more low-fat foods.

Here's a checklist for you and the person in your care:

- Be realistic. Make small changes over time. Small steps can work better than giant leaps.

- Be daring and try new foods.

- Be flexible. Balance food intake with physical activity over several days. Don't focus on just one meal or one day.

- Be sensible and practice not overdoing it.

- Be active and choose activities that you enjoy and that fit into the rest of your life.

Special Needs and Considerations

Good nutrition is necessary for everyone, but sometimes things can get in the way of eating right. Ask the nurse, doctor, or pharmacist if any of the medications the person in your care is taking have possible side effects that can interfere with appetite or affect the absorption of important vitamins and minerals.

Changes in mobility. If eating habits remain the same while activity drops off, ***weight gain*** can result. Added weight can increase fatigue, further limit mobility, put a strain on the respiratory and circulatory systems (lungs, heart, blood, blood vessels), and increase the risk of other chronic illnesses. Ask a registered dietitian to recommend an ideal weight and reasonable daily calorie intake to maintain that weight. To get weight under control, pair exercise with healthy eating.

Additionally, inadequate physical activity, lack of weight-bearing exercise, and an increasingly sedentary lifestyle can result from changes in mobility that can contribute to the risk of developing ***osteoporosis*** (see p. 179)—a condition where bones can become thin and fragile. While building strong bones started early in childhood, keeping them healthy as we grow older requires attention and care. Good nutrition—particularly daily sources of calcium—is important for maintaining bone health.

- Choose nonfat or low-fat dairy products often.

- Eat any type of fish with edible bones,

- Choose dark-green vegetables like kale, broccoli, turnip greens, and mustard greens. The calcium in these veggies is better absorbed than the calcium found in spinach, rhubarb, beet greens, and almonds.

- Calcium-fortified tofu, soymilk, orange juice, breads, and cereals are excellent staples. Check the food labels to see just how much calcium has been added.

- Vitamin D also plays an important role in bone health by helping with the calcium absorption. Our bodies can make vitamin D with just 15–20 minutes of skin exposure to the sun each day. Vitamin D can also be found fortified in foods that contain calcium. Be careful with supplementation because vitamin D is stored in the body and can be toxic in relatively low amounts (>2,000 i.u./day)

Eating and emotions. Depression can affect people's appetite in different ways. Many people turn to certain foods for comfort when they are depressed. These may be old favorites from childhood—a scoop of mashed potatoes, macaroni and cheese, a bowl of rice pudding. The danger is in overdoing it. These foods are often high in fat, sugar, and calories that can easily add up. On the other hand, some people lose their appetite when they are depressed. Eating with others can help you and the person in your care stay connected. Remember also that being physically active can help decrease the symptoms of depression.

Bladder problems are another issue. Quite often, fear of having to go to the bathroom frequently or loss of bladder control causes a person to limit fluids. This can cause other problems such as dehydration, dry mouth, difficulty swallowing, loss of appetite, and constipation. Find ways to fit in fluids.

- To avoid sleep disturbance, do not drink fluid late at night (after 6 pm).

- Take water breaks during the day.

- Have a beverage with meals.

- "Water down" your meals and snacks.

- Take a drink when you pass a water fountain.

- Travel with your own personal supply of bottled water.

Bowel management often involves preventing constipation. Fiber counts . . . add it up. Fiber is found in cereal, grains, nuts, seeds, vegetables, and fruit. It is not completely digested (broken down) or absorbed (taken in) by the body. A diet rich in fiber (about 25 to 30 grams each day) along with adequate fluid intake and physical activity can help promote good bowel function. Fiber can also provide a sense of fullness, which helps in managing how much one eats.

People with liver disease usually have problems with diarrhea due to changes in absorption. Lactulose can also cause diarrhea.

Careful Food Preparation

People with chronic disease are susceptible to illness from unsafe food, so be extra careful when preparing their meals.

- Wash your own hands and the hands of the person in your care with antibacterial soap before preparing or serving food.

- Dry hands with a paper towel.

- Disinfect the sink and kitchen counters with a solution of 1 teaspoon chlorine bleach per liter of water. (Save the solution for just one week because it loses strength.)

- Air drying dishes is more sanitary than using a dish towel.

- Check expiration dates carefully, and discard all meats that are past the expiration date on the label.

- Cook all red meat and fish thoroughly. Avoid red meat as much as possible.

- Cook hamburgers or chopped meat to an internal temperature of 160° F. (There is much less chance of being infected by a solid piece of meat like a steak or roast because bacteria collects only on the outside of those cuts.)

- Cook meat at least at an oven temperature of 300° F.

- Keep hot foods hot at 140° F or more and cold foods at 40° F or colder.

- Keep the refrigerator below 41° F.

- Cook eggs until the yolks are no longer runny.

- Don't serve raw eggs in milk shakes or other drinks.

- Don't serve oysters, clams, or shellfish raw.

- Wash all fruits and vegetables thoroughly.

- Avoid unpasteurized milk and cider.

 If the water temperature is set too low, the dishwasher will not sterilize the dishes.

Exercise as Part of Life

Physical activity and good nutrition are perfect partners in good health. This winning combination finds a balance between what one eats and one's daily activities. Together they help in managing weight and providing energy. Care receivers with advanced liver disease often end up with muscle wasting. It is important that these people exercise to preserve muscle mass.

Physical activity not only burns calories, but it can also help the person in your care by doing the following:

- Make the most of muscle strength, or even build strength, depending on the program.

- Slowly increase the ability to do more for longer periods of time.

- Increase range of motion and joint flexibility (the ability to move easily).

- Strengthen the heart.

- Decrease feelings of fatigue.

- Decrease symptoms of depression.

- Maintain regular bowel and bladder functions.

- Cut down on the risk of skin breakdown and irritation.

- Protect weight-bearing bone mass (spine, hips, legs).

Good physical fitness is made up of three types of exercise: stretching, strengthening, and aerobics. Each is important by itself, but together they can help the person in your care remain active as long as possible. This will help the person deal better with the changes illness may bring.

A person should always stretch before exercise. This warms the muscles, helps prevent stiffness, and improves flexibility and balance. The person should work at his or her own pace, even if it seems very slow. Encourage the person in your care, even if the exercises seem difficult at first. Watch for signs of fatigue. Always cool down after exercise.

Stretching

Regular *s-t-r-e-t-c-h-i-n-g* is the first step, and it can be one of the most enjoyable. Stretching helps muscle rigidity (stiffness). It also helps muscles and joints stay flexible (able to bend). People who are more flexible have an easier time with everyday movement. Stretching can also help with muscle cramps.

Stretching increases range of motion of joints and helps with good posture. It protects against muscle strains or sprains, improves circulation, and releases muscle tension.

Do's and Don'ts of Stretching

- **DO** stretch to the point of a gentle pull.

- **DON'T** stretch to the point of pain.

- **DON'T** bounce while stretching.

- **DON'T** hold the breath during a stretch. Breathe evenly in and out during each stretch.

- **DON'T** compare yourself to others.

Stretching can be done at any time. The person in your care can start the day by stretching before getting out of bed. Have the person stretch throughout the day, while watching television or riding in a car.

Aerobic activities raise the heart rate and breathing, and promote cardiovascular (heart and lung) fitness. Other activities develop strength and flexibility. For example, lifting weights develops strength and can help maintain good bone health. Activities like yoga and gentle stretching can improve flexibility.

Some key points to remember:

- You and the person in your care should talk with the doctor about exercise, target weight, and special needs. If possible, get a referral to a physical therapist to help begin the program.

- An exercise program needs to match the abilities and limitations of the individual. A physical therapist can design a well-balanced exercise program for those who need more help. With some changes, people at all levels of disability can enjoy the benefits of exercise.

- The person in your care should commit to doing what he or she can do on a consistent basis. Choosing activities you both enjoy will help you stick to your fitness plan.

- Start slowly. If the person in your care hasn't been active, begin at a low level of intensity for short periods. Alternate brief periods of exercise with periods of rest until the person in your care begins to build up endurance. Gradually increase how hard you are exercising and the length of time you are doing it.

- Join a group! Exercising with others may give you the motivation and support to keep going.

NOTE A person begins to get aerobic benefit from exercise when his heart rate hits 50 percent of its maximum. No one should exceed 80 percent of his maximum heart rate during exercise.

To figure maximum heart rate, subtract age from 220. For example, maximum heart rate for a 60-year-old person is 160. For aerobic benefit, he must get the heart rate up to 80 beats per minute and should not exceed 130 beats per minute.

For many care receivers, because of age or level of debility, the standard exercise prescription of 30 minutes most days of the week is simply not possible. So understand from the beginning that the care receiver's activity level won't look like a healthy person's.

Moving in Water

Water therapy is a time-tested form of healing. It is also a safe way for a person with a disability to exercise because there is no danger of falling. Floating in water allows easy movement and little strain on joints and muscles.

Using a kickboard or simply walking in place in water may produce aerobic benefit. Water also resists movement so it produces increased heart rate in less time. Water can also be a good place to exercise for those with balance problems. Talk to a physical therapist about whether a water aerobics class might be appropriate for the person in your care.

Tip YMCAs often offer water aerobics classes that your care receiver might participate in.

Moving on Land

Aerobic exercise on land for the elderly or people with disabilities is more problematic. A readily available option is chair exercises. These allow the person to remain seated while providing aerobic benefit.

Tip There are several DVD and video products that have complete workouts. In your search engine, type "chair exercises" or "chair dancing."

Weight Training

Muscles often weaken as a result of not being used. Weight training can be a major help in restoring these muscles. Recent research indicates that targeted strength training in patients with muscle weakness significantly increased muscle power without any negative effects.

People with liver disease should avoid lifting heavy weights (more than 5–10 lbs) because they can have varicose veins in the esophagus and weight lifting increases the chance that these veins will bleed.

Do not take the person in your care to the weight room and just leave her there. She will need supervision and instruction. Most physical trainers do not have enough special training to work with people with disabilities, but increasingly it is possible to find special needs strength trainers who may be able to help. For a basic special needs weight workout, visit **www.progressiverecovery.com.**

Tip To improve balance at home, bring a chair to the corner of a room. While the care receiver stands in the corner, she can hold on to the back of the chair and practice moving shoulders and hips together from side to side and then forward and backward.

Tai Chi

Tai chi is a slow, flowing form of ancient Chinese exercise. It aids in flexibility, balance, and relaxation. Several forms of tai chi can be done by anyone regardless of age or physical condition. Classes are often offered at fitness centers, senior centers, and community recreation centers. Speak with the instructor to learn if the type of tai chi he or she teaches is best for the person in your care. Tai chi programs are also available on videotape at a variety of retail stores.

Yoga

Yoga is a form of exercise that can be very helpful for persons with chronic illness. It increases flexibility, relaxation, and awareness of breathing and posture. Yoga also can reduce stress. Yoga is self-paced, which means that people can do the poses in their own way and hold the pose for as long as they are comfortable. Yoga can even be done in a chair.

It is important to contact the instructor prior to beginning a class. Generally, a beginner class or a class for those with special needs is a good place for your care receiver to start.

Tip If the person in your care has significant balance impairment, Tai Chi and yoga moves from a chair may be necessary.

Creative Expression

Creative expression can provide movement and physical activity. Painting on an easel with large, strong strokes stretches the arms and shoulders. "Conducting" the music of a favorite symphony or opera has shown to have a strengthening and aerobic benefit. Singing alone or in a choral group promotes the deep breathing needed for louder speech. Encourage the person in your care to seek creative outlets that fit their talents and abilities.

Remember, before starting any type of workout routine, get advice from your physician. Start slowly with only moderate effort. Give the care receiver time to build strength and stamina. Any amount of exercise helps reduce risk, and the benefits of exercise are cumulative, so find a way to make it easy to get exercise, that way he or she is more likely to do it. Exercise is a particularly effective way to reduce depression.

And finally, everything said here about the benefits of aerobic exercise and weight training also applies to the caregiver. *You* need exercise as much as the person in your care. Find a way to make it part of most days.

Motivation

Motivation is the #1 factor determining whether people change their lifestyles or fail to follow their exercise and diet prescriptions. While motivation is an inside job, the caregiver has a part to play. Do what you can to make exercise fun. Make the new diet an experiment. If you make either diet or exercise too important, any failure becomes that much more significant. Keep it light-hearted, maintain a sense of humor, and join in as much as possible.

No single day of exercise or eating right makes much of a difference in your or your care receiver's health, but 30 days do. Sixty days makes even more of an impact; a year's worth of a new lifestyle will provide remarkable shifts of biomarkers (a specific physical trait used to measure the effects or progress of a disease or condition; thinning hair is an example of a biomarker for aging), mood, and self-esteem. People who take up the challenge presented by diet and exercise prescriptions make huge strides in their physical and emotional recovery; imagine what it does to their independence.

Exercise and the Daily Routine

A good exercise regimen can help a person maintain mobility.

Some persons may not be able to follow an exercise program due to changes in their physical ability. It may be better for those people to fit exercises and stretching into the daily routine:

- Find a simple activity that the person enjoys, such as walking, gardening, housekeeping, or swimming. As caregiver, you can try to make some of these activities part of the daily routine.

- Sitting and reaching in different directions can stretch the arms and trunk.

- Household chores such as folding laundry, dusting, wiping dishes, or helping with food preparation provide gentle exercise.

- Simple games like balloon volleyball, playing catch with a large, soft ball or blowing soap bubbles are an enjoyable way to get exercise.

- Music creates movement such as marching or dancing. If balance is a problem, try chair dancing. "Conducting" to the beat of up-tempo music provides upper body exercise and good emotional therapy!

- Perform a few extra arm and leg motions during dressing tasks.

A physical therapist can suggest exercises and stretches that will suit the person in your care. Therapists can also provide ways to improve walking and balance, if necessary.

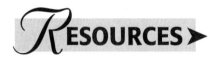

RESOURCES ➤

American Dietetic Association
(800) 366-1655
Call weekdays 10:00 a.m. to 5:00 p.m. EST to locate a registered dietitian in your area.

Area Agency on Aging or the Cooperative Extension Service
Your local office offers free counseling by a registered dietitian.

Meals-on-Wheels
Can provide nutritious meals delivered to the home.

MyPyramid

www.mypyramid.gov
This replaces the old Food Guide Pyramid. It is a very interactive site to help people make healthy choices consistent with the latest Dietary Guidelines for Americans.

The National Sports Center for the Disabled (NSCD)

P.O. Box 1290
Winter Park, CO 80482
(970) 726-1540
www.nscd.org
E-mail: info@nscd.org
NSCD is a nonprofit corporation that offers winter and summer recreation. Winter sports include snow skiing, snowshoeing, and cross-country skiing. Summer recreation activities include fishing, hiking, rock climbing, whitewater rafting, camping, mountain biking, sailing, therapeutic horseback riding, and a baseball camp.

Publication

A Modification of the Rules of Golf for Golfers with Disabilities
United States Golf Association
P.O. Box 708
Far Hills, NJ 07931-0708
(908) 234-2300
www.usga.org/playing/rules/golfers_with_disabilities.html
Online publication contains permissible modifications to the rules of golf for players with a disability.

If you don't have access to the Internet, ask your local library to help you locate a Web site.

Emergencies

Emergencies

*E*mergency situations are common when caring for a person with chronic illness. Many injuries can be avoided through preventive measures (📖 see **Preparing the Home, p. 88**). When a crisis does occur, use common sense, stay calm, and realize that you can help.

NOTE Make sure 911 is posted on your phone or ideally is on speed-dial. Keep written driving instructions near the phone for how to get to your house. If you have a speakerphone, use the speaker when talking to the dispatcher. This way, you can follow the dispatcher's instructions while attending to the emergency.

When to Call for an Ambulance

Call for an ambulance if a person—

- is vomiting blood or is bleeding from the rectum

- becomes disoriented and confused

- has severe abdominal pain or pressure that does not go away

- has a high fever (>101° F) that is not brought down with medication or has a low body temperature (<94° F)

- becomes unconscious

- has chest pain or pressure

- has trouble breathing

- has no signs of breathing (no movement or response to touch or voice)

- has fallen and may have broken bones

- has had a seizure

- has a severe headache and slurred speech

OR

- if moving the person could cause further injury

- if traffic or distance would cause a life-threatening delay in getting to the hospital

- if the person is too heavy for you to lift or help

Ambulance service is expensive and may not be covered by insurance. Use it when you believe there is an emergency.

In an emergency:

Step 1: Call 911.
Step 2: Care for the victim.

Also call 911 for emergencies involving fire, explosion, poisonous gas, fallen electrical wires, overdose of medicine or other life-threatening situations.

NOTE If the person in your care has signed a Do Not Resuscitate (DNR) order, have it available to show the paramedics. Otherwise, they are required to initiate resuscitation (reviving the person). The order must go with the patient. The Do Not Resuscitate order must be with the patient at all times.

In the Emergency Room

Bring to the emergency room—

- insurance policy numbers

- a list of medical problems

- all medications currently being taken by the patient

- the personal physician's name, phone number

- the liver transplant center's name, phone number and contact person

- the name and number of a relative or friend of the person in your care

Before leaving the emergency room, be sure you understand the instructions for care. If the patient is listed for a liver transplantation, call the person's primary care doctor and the transplant center as soon as possible. Let them know about the emergency room care.

We strongly suggest that you take a course in CPR from your local American Red Cross, hospital, or other agency.

Bleeding

Bleeding Due to End-Stage Liver Disease

People with end-stage liver disease are prone to bleeding either from the upper gastrointestinal (GI) tract (esophagus, stomach) or the lower GI tract (rectum).

Upper GI bleeding can present either as vomiting bright red blood or dark vomit that looks like dried up coffee grounds or dark black stool. If the person in your care develops a sudden episode of vomiting blood, coffee-ground vomit, or bright red blood from the rectum, CALL 911 IMMEDIATELY. This is a life-threatening problem and requires emergent medical attention. After calling 911, lay him on his side to prevent aspiration.

If the person in your care has continuous dark black stool with complaints of dizziness or weakness then call 911.

Prevention

• Make sure the person in your care is taking her beta-blocker (propranolol, nadolol) and proton pump inhibitor (Nexium, Protonix, Aciphex) regularly if prescribed by the physician.

• Update her endoscopy (procedure where a camera is placed down the patient's throat to check for varicose veins in the food pipe) regularly.

Bleeding Not from the GI Tract

People with end-stage liver disease have clotting problems so they are more likely to bleed spontaneously. If they bleed, it may be hard to control.

If someone is bleeding heavily, protect yourself with rubber gloves, plastic wrap, or layers of cloth. Then—

1. Apply direct pressure over the wound with a clean cloth.

2. Apply another clean cloth on top of the blood-soaked cloth, keeping the pressure firm.

3. If no bones are broken, elevate (raise) the injured limb to decrease blood flow.

4. Call 911 for an ambulance.

5. Apply a bandage snugly over the dressing.

6. Wash your hands with soap and water as soon as possible after providing care.

7. Avoid contact with blood-soaked objects.

Confusion and Disorientation with End-Stage Liver Disease

If the person in your care becomes disoriented or confused, it can mean the following things:

- worsening encephalopathy (confusion associated with end stage liver disease)

- dehydration

- infection

Call 911, and contact the care receiver's liver transplant team or liver doctor.

Prevention

- Give the person in your care lactulose (sweet syrup pre-scribed by physician) regularly and adjust to have 3–4 soft, pudding-like bowel movements per day. This is the only medication you can adjust on your own.

- Make sure the person in your care is well hydrated and not having diarrhea from the lactulose since this can induce dehydration and lead to confusion.

- Decrease the amount of red meat the person in your care eats.

> *Tip*
>
> Diarrhea can lead to dehydration, which can increase confusion. It is very important that the caregiver pay attention to the number of bowel movements the care receiver has each day and adjust the lactulose daily.

Shock

Shock may be associated with heavy bleeding, hives, shortness of breath, dizziness, swelling, thirst, and chest pain. The signs of shock are:

- restlessness and irritability

- confusion, altered consciousness

- pale, cool, moist skin

- rapid breathing and weakness

If these signs are present—

1. Have the person lie down.

2. Control any bleeding.

3. Keep the person warm.

4. Elevate the legs about 12 to 14 inches unless the neck or back has been injured.

5. Do not give the person anything to eat or drink.

6. Call 911.

Chest Pain

Any chest pain that lasts more than a few minutes is related to the heart until proven otherwise. CALL 911 IMMEDIATELY. Don't wait to see if it goes away. Danger signs include—

- pain radiating from the chest down the arms, up the neck to the jaw, and into the back

- crushing, squeezing chest pain or heavy pressure in the chest

- shortness of breath, sweating, nausea and vomiting, weakness

- bluish, pale skin

- skin that is moist

- excessive perspiration

If the person is unresponsive (no movement or response to touch or voice), **call 911**. Be prepared to give Rescue Breathing and start CPR as instructed in CPR class.

Abdominal Pain or Pressure

Sudden abdominal pain or pressure in a person with end-stage liver disease can be a sign of a serious and life-threatening infection or a possible blood clot in the abdomen.

CALL 911, and contact the liver transplant team or liver doctor.

Prevention

If the person in your care was put on an antibiotic due to a history of prior infection (spontaneous bacterial peritonitis), make sure he takes the medication regularly. Most commonly used antibiotics are norfloxacin or bactrim.

Falls and Related Injuries

Preventive measures include—

- staying in when it is rainy or icy outside

- having regular vision screening check-ups for correct eye glasses

- using separate reading glasses and other regular glasses if bifocals make it difficult to see the floor

- being cautious when walking on wet floors

- wearing good foot support when walking

- being aware that new shoes are slippery and crepe-soled shoes can cause the toe to catch

- having foot pain problems corrected

- keeping toenails trimmed and feet healthy for good balance

Use walkers or cane if needed.

Fainting

Fainting can be caused by—

- a heart attack

- medications

- low blood sugar

- standing up quickly

- straining to have a bowel movement

- dehydration / hepatic encephalopathy

- seizure

To some extent, fainting can be prevented.

- Ask the doctor if medications that do not cause fainting can be prescribed.

- Monitor blood sugar levels.

- Avoid constipation.

- Avoid dehydration.

- Do not let the person stand up or sit up too rapidly.

 Tip

Patients on certain medicines such as propanolol or nadolol can have decreased heart rate and/or decreased blood pressure. Rapid movement can induce dizziness in these patients. Have them sit up for few minutes before standing up from a lying down position.

If a fainting spell occurs:

1. Do not try to place the person in a sitting position. Instead, immediately lay him down flat.

2. Check the person's airway, breathing, and pulse.

3. Turn the person on his side.

4. Elevate the legs.

5. Cover him with a blanket if the room or floor is cold.

6. Do not give fluids.

7. Call 911 if person is having difficulty breathing, not breathing, or not responding to your voice and touch.

8. If not breathing, be prepared to give Rescue Breathing and start CPR as instructed in CPR class.

Poisons

If you suspect poisoning, immediately take these steps:

1. Determine **what** was swallowed, **how much,** and at **what time.**

2. Check the person's airway. (Are there signs of breathing, coughing, moving?)

3. Contact the nearest Poison Control Center or call 911 for treatment; have the container of the suspected poison at hand.

4. Follow up with the doctor.

5. If not breathing (no movement or response to touch or voice) call 911 and be prepared to give Rescue Breathing and start CPR as instructed in CPR class.

Seizures

A seizure usually lasts from 1 to 5 minutes. If it lasts longer than you are comfortable with or more than 7 minutes, call 911 for an ambulance.

1. Remove all objects that might cause the person to injure himself.

2. Place pillows and blankets around him to protect him.

3. Do not hold or restrain the person.

4. Do not place anything in the person's mouth.

5. Always check for **breathing** and **signs of circulation** after the seizure stops.

6. Reassure and comfort the person.

7. If the person is unresponsive (no movement or response to touch or voice), call 911 and be prepared to give Rescue Breathing (1 breath every 5–6 seconds) and start CPR as instructed in CPR class.

Stroke

Strokes occur when the blood flow to the brain is interrupted by a clogged or burst blood vessel. Strokes cannot always be prevented, but the chances of their occurring can be lessened through—

• a balanced diet

• avoidance of stress

• periodic checkups

• regular exercise

• regular use of a prescribed blood pressure medicine

Suspect a stroke when the person in your care—

• has a sudden and severe headache

• does not respond to simple statements

• has a seizure

- is suddenly incontinent (unable to control bladder and bowel)

- has paralysis (cannot move) in an arm or leg

- cannot grip equally with both hands

- appears droopy on one side of the face

- has slurred speech or blurred vision

- is confused

- has an unsteady gait

- has trouble swallowing

- has loss of balance or coordination when combined with one of the other signs

The chance of recovery from a stroke is greatly increased if the person has immediate help.

1. Keep the person in the position you found him in.

2. Reassure him and keep him calm.

3. If he has trouble breathing, open his airway, tilt his head, and lift his chin.

4. Call 911. Get the person to medical care as soon as possible.

5. If the person is not breathing, give 2 Rescue Breaths.

6. If breathing resumes, place the person on one side to prevent choking. This also helps keep the tongue out of the airway.

7. If the person is unresponsive (no movement or response to touch or voice), be prepared to give Rescue Breathing and start CPR as instructed in CPR class.

Checklist Home First Aid Kit

Buy or make a home first-aid kit. Note on the box the date when the item was purchased. Check and replenish your supplies at least once a year. These should include the following:

✓ *antibiotic ointment*

✓ *Band-Aids®*

✓ *disinfectant for cleaning wounds*

✓ *disposable gloves*

✓ *emergency telephone numbers*

✓ *eye pads*

✓ *instant ice packs*

✓ *list of current medications*

✓ *pocket mask/face mask*

✓ *rolled gauze and elastic bandages*

✓ *scissors*

✓ *sterile gauze bandages (nonstick 4"×4")*

✓ *syrup of ipecac*

✓ *thermometer*

✓ *tongue depressors*

✓ *3-ounce rubber bulb to rinse out wounds*

✓ *triangle bandage*

✓ *tweezers and needle*

Part Three: Additional Resources

Part 3 ✣ Additional Resources

Common Abbreviations

Acute MI – heart attack

ADA – Americans with Disabilities Act

ADL – activities of daily living

AFO – ankle-foot orthosis

ALF – assisted living facility

ASHD – arteriosclerotic heart disease

BC – blood culture

BID – 2 times per day (approximately 8 and 8 as medication times)

BP – blood pressure

BRP – bathroom privileges

BS – blood sugar

C&S – culture and sensitivity

CA – cancer/carcinoma

CABG – coronary artery bypass graft

CBC – complete blood count

CCU – coronary care unit

CHF – congestive heart failure

CNS – central nervous system

COPD – chronic obstructive pulmonary disease

CPR – cardiopulmonary resuscitation

CSF – cerebrospinal fluid

CVA – cerebral vascular

CVD – cerebral vascular disease

DM – diabetes mellitus

DME – durable medical equipment

DNR – do not resuscitate

DRG – diagnosis related group

Dx – diagnosis

ED – emergency department

EEG – electroencephalogram recording of the brain's electrical activity

EKG/ECG – electrocardiogram recording of the heart's electrical activity

EP – evoked potential

ESLD – End-Stage Liver Disease

FBS – fasting blood sugar, or the amount of glucose in the blood when a person has not eaten for 12 hours

FX – fracture

GTT – glucose tolerance test to determine a person's ability to metabolize glucose

HBV – hepatitis B virus

HC – home care

HCV – Hepatitis C Virus

HHA – a home health agency providing home health services

HS – hour of sleep (medication time)

I&O – record of food and liquid taken in and waste eliminated

ICU – intensive care unit for special monitoring of the acutely ill

IV – intravenous line to drip fluids and blood products into the bloodstream

LOC – loss of consciousness

MCD – Medicaid

MCR – Medicare

MELD – Model for End-Stage Liver Disease

MRI – magnetic resonance imaging

Neuro – neurologist

NPO – nothing by mouth

NSAID – nonsteroid antiinflammatory drug.

OBS – organic brain syndrome, an injury or disorder that interferes with normal brain function

OR – operating room

OT – occupational therapy or occupational therapist

PO – by mouth

Psych – psychologist

PT – physical therapy or physical therapist

QID – 4 times per day (approximately 9–1–5–9 as medication times)

RBC – red blood count

RN – Registered Nurse

ROM – range of motion

RR – respiratory rate

RT – recreational therapy

Rx – prescription

SLP – speech-language pathologist

SNF – skilled nursing facility

SOB – shortness of breath

SS or SSA – Social Security or Social Security Administration

SSI/SSDI – supplemental security income or disability income

ST – Speech therapist or speech therapy

Sx – symptoms

TIA – transient ischemic attack

TID – 3 times per day (approximately 9–1–6 as medication times)

TPN – total parenteral nutrition

TPR – temperature, pulse, respiration

TX – treatment

U/A – urine analysis

VEP – visual evoked potential

VNS – visiting nurse service

WBC – white blood count

Common Specialists

Allergist/Immunologist
Disorders of the immune system

Anesthesiologist
Pain relief during and after surgery

Audiologist
Hearing disorders

Cardiologist
Conditions of the heart, lungs, and blood vessels

Chiropodist
Minor foot ailments such as corns and bunions

Colon and Rectal Surgeon
Diseases of the intestinal tract

Dentist
Teeth and gums

Dermatologist
Skin, hair, and nails

Endocrinologist
Hormonal problems including thyroid disorders

Forensic Psychiatrist
Behavior assessment for legal purposes

Gastroenterologist
Digestive system, stomach, bowels, and gallbladder

Geriatric Psychiatrist
Emotional disorders of elderly persons

Geriatrician
Disorders common to elderly persons

Gynecologist
Female reproductive system

Hematologist
Diseases of the blood, spleen, and lymph glands

Hepatologist
Specialist in liver disease

Internist
Primary care of common illnesses, both long term and emergency

Nephrologist
Kidney diseases and disorders

Neurologist
Brain and nervous system disorders

Nurse Practitioner
Provides preventive and medical health care in association with a physician

Oncologist
All cancers

Ophthalmologist
Care and surgery of the eyes

Optician
Fitting and making of eyeglasses and contact lenses

Optometrist
Basic eye care

Oral Maxillofacial Surgeon
Surgery involving the teeth, gums, and jaw

Orthopedist
Surgery involving joints, bones, and muscles

Orthotist
Nonmedical specialist in the measurement, sizing, and preparation of foot padding pieces

Osteopath (DO)
General medicine with emphasis on the promotion of health through the hands-on manipulation of the muscles, tendons, and joints

Otolaryngologist
Head and neck surgeon

Pharmacist
Medications specialist; provider of physician and patient education

Physician assistant
Provides preventive and medical health care in association with a physician

Podiatrist
Foot care

Psychiatrist (MD)
Emotional, mental, or addictive disorders

Psychologist (MA or PhD)
Assessment and care of emotional or mental disorders

Pulmonologist
Diseases of lungs and airways

Rheumatologist
Diseases of joints and connective tissue (arthritis)

Urologist
Urinary system and the male reproductive system

Caregiver Organizations

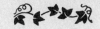

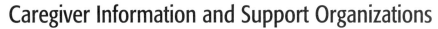

Caregiver Information and Support Organizations

. . . And Thou Shalt Honor
http://www.thoushalthonor.org/
The site for the acclaimed PBS caregiving documentary . . . And Thou Shalt Honor provides a variety of caregiving tools and resources.

Everyday Warriors
www.everydaywarriors.com
This site features numerous articles of interest to caregivers of all ages. Visit "Ask the Caregiver Coach," and "Caregivers Sound Off."

FamilyCare America, Inc.
1004 N. Thompson St., Suite 205
Richmond, VA 23230
(804) 342-2200
www.FamilyCareAmerica.com
FamilyCare America is dedicated to improving the lives of caregivers of the elderly, disabled, and chronically ill by creating a highly accessible resource where caregivers can:

- *better learn the process of caregiving*
- *receive help in managing their fears and concerns*
- *obtain resources for help with all aspects of caregiving*

Caregiver Organizations

Family Caregivers Alliance
690 Market Street, Suite 600
San Francisco, CA 94104
(800) 445-8106; 415-434-3388 Fax: (415) 434-3508
www.caregiver.org
E-mail: info@caregiver.org
Resource center for caregivers of people with chronic disabling conditions. The Web site provides information on services and programs in education, research, and advocacy.

National Alliance for Caregiving
4720 Montgomery Lane, 5th Floor
Bethesda, MD 20814
www.caregiving.org
The Alliance is a non-profit coalition of national organizations focusing on issues of family caregiving.

National Family Caregivers Association
10400 Connecticut Avenue, Suite 500
Kensington, MD 20895
(800) 896-3650
www.thefamilycaregiver.org
The Association supports, empowers, educates, and speaks up for the more than 50 million Americans who care for a chronically ill, aged, or disabled person.

National Quality Caregiving Coalition
750 First Street, NE
Washington, DC 20002-4242
(202) 336-5606
www.nqcc-rci.org
The NQCC is a coalition of national associations, groups, and individuals with interests in and active agendas that promote caregiving across all ages and disabilities throughout the lifespan.

Well Spouse Association
63 West Main Street—Suite H
Freehold, NJ 07728
(800) 838-0879
www.wellspouse.org
E-mail: info@wellspouse.org
A national, not-for-profit membership organization that gives support to wives, husbands, and partners of the chronically ill and/or disabled.

Insurance Issues

Geriatric Care Managers
National Association of Geriatric Care Managers
http://www.caremanager.org/

Medicare
http://www.medicare.gov/
General information about Medicare.

Medicare Rights Center
www.medicarerights.org
Having difficulties dealing with the health insurance maze? For those who have questions or problems regarding coverage, this not-for-profit, non-governmental website can provide some answers and suggestions.

International Caregiver Information and Support Organizations

AUSTRALIA

Carers Australia
www.carersaustralia.com.au
(800) 242-636

Carers Australia represents the needs and interests of caregivers at the national level by

- *Advocating for carers' needs and interests in the public arena.*

- *Influencing government and stakeholder policies and programs at the national level through conducting research and pilot projects, giving presentations, and participating in a wide range of inquiries, reviews, and policy forums.*

- *Networking and forming strategic partnerships with other organizations to achieve positive outcomes for carers.*

- *Providing carers with information and education resources, undertaking community activities to raise awareness, and coordinating and facilitating joint work between the state and territory organizations on matters of national significance.*

CANADA

Canadian Caregiver Coalition

www.ccc-ccan.ca
The Canadian Caregivers Coalition helps identify and respond to the needs of caregivers in Canada. Links to organizations helpful to caregivers.

Caregiver Network, Inc.

(416) 323-1090
www.caregiver.on.ca
Based in Toronto, Canada, CNI's goal is to be a national single-information source to make your life as a caregiver easier.

UNITED KINGDOM

Carers UK

www.carersuk.org
The leading campaigning, policy, and information organization for carers; membership organization, led and set up by carers in 1965 to have a voice and to win the recognition and support that carers deserve.

Glossary

A

Activities of daily living (ADL): personal hygiene, bathing, dressing, grooming, toileting, feeding, and transferring

Acute: state of illness that comes on suddenly and may be of short duration

Alcoholic stool: pale whitish-color stool, can be due to liver disease

Advance directive: a legal document that states a person's health care preferences in writing while that person is competent and able to make such decisions

Ambulatory: able to walk with little or no assistance

Amnesia: complete or partial loss of memory

Analgesics: medications used to relieve pain

Antibiotics: a group of drugs used to combat infection

Anxiety: a state of discomfort, dread, and foreboding with physical symptoms such as rapid breathing and heart rate, tension, jitteriness, and muscle aches

Apathy: a condition in which the person shows little or no emotion

Artificial life-support systems: the use of respirators, tube feeding, intravenous (IV) feeding, and other means to replace natural and vital functions, such as breathing, eating, and drinking

Ascites: water in the abdomen

Assessment: the process of analyzing a person's condition

Assistive devices: any tools that are designed, fabricated, and/or adapted to assist a person in performing a particular task, e.g., cane, walker, shower chair

Asterixis: a physical finding in patients with cirrhosis that represents confusion manifesting as flapping of both hands when stretched out straight.

Atrophy: the wasting away of muscles or brain tissue

ॐ B

Bedpan: a container into which a person urinates and defecates while in bed

Bilirubin: break-down of red blood cells, processed by liver and secreted out of the body through stool and urine

Blood pressure: the pressure of the blood on the walls of the blood vessels and arteries

Body mechanics: proper use and positioning of the body to do work and avoid strain and injury

ॐ C

Calorie: the measure of the energy the body gets from various foods

Catheter: a rubber tube for collecting urine from a person who has become incontinent

Chronic: refers to a state or condition that lasts 6 months or longer

Cirrhosis: a lot of scar tissue replacing normal cells in the liver leading to liver failure

Cognition: high-level functions carried out by the human brain, including comprehension and use of speech, visual perception and construction, calculation ability, attention (information processing), memory, and executive functions such as planning, problem-solving, and self-monitoring

Cognitive rehabilitation: techniques used to improve the functioning of individuals whose cognition is impaired because of physical trauma or disease

Colostomy: a temporary or permanent surgical procedure that creates an artificial opening through the abdominal wall into a part of the large bowel through which feces can leave the body

Conservator: a person given the power to take over and protect the interests of one who is incompetent

Constipation: difficulty having bowel movements

ॐ D

Decubitus ulcer: pressure sore; bedsore

Defecate: to have a bowel movement

Defibrillator: a device that uses an electrical current to restore or regulate a stopped or disorganized heartbeat

Dehydration: loss of normal body fluid, sometimes caused by vomiting and severe diarrhea

Delusions: beliefs that are firmly held despite proof that they are false

Dementia: a progressive decline in mental functions

Depression: a psychiatric condition that can be moderate or severe and cause feelings of sadness and emptiness

Diuretics: drugs that help the body get rid of fluids

Durable Power of Attorney: a legal document that authorizes another to act as one's agent and is "durable" because it remains in effect in case the person becomes disabled or mentally incompetent

Durable Power of Attorney for Health Care Decisions: a legal document that lets a person name someone else to make health care decisions after the person has become disabled or mentally incompetent and is unable to make those decisions

Dysphagia: difficulty with or abnormal swallowing

E

Edema: an abnormal swelling in legs, ankles, hands, or abdomen that occurs because the body is retaining fluids

Encephalopathy: confusion due to increase in ammonia level in a patient with cirrhosis

Esophagus: food pipe connecting the mouth to the stomach

Esophageal varices: varicose veins in the esophagus that may enlarge with cirrhosis and may rupture

Estate planning: a process of planning for the present and future use of a person's assets

F

Foot drop: a condition of weakness in the muscles of the foot and ankle, caused by poor nerve conduction, which interferes with a person's ability to flex the ankle and walk with a normal heel–toe pattern; the toes touch the ground before the heel, causing the person to trip or lose balance

G

Gait: the manner in which a person walks

Guardian: the one who is designated to have protective care of another person or of that person's property

H

Hallucination: false perceptions of things that are not really there
Heimlich maneuver: a method for clearing the airway of a choking person
Hematochezia: bright red blood in the stool
Hepatocelluar carcinoma (HCC): primary liver cancer
Hospice: a program that allows a dying person to remain at home while receiving professionally supervised care

I

Incontinence: involuntary discharge of urine or feces
Intravenous (IV): the delivery of fluids, medications, or nutrients into a vein

J

Jaundice: yellowing of the skin and eyes due to increase in bilirubin

L

Laxative: a substance taken to increase bowel movements and prevent constipation

M

Mechanical lift: a machine used to lift a person from one place to another
Medic-Alert®: bracelet identification system linked to a 24-hour service that provides full information in the case of an emergency
Medicaid: a public health program that uses state and federal funds to pay certain medical and hospital expenses of those having low income or no income, with benefits that vary from state to state
Medicare: the federal health insurance program for people 65 or older and for certain people under 65 who are disabled
Melena: dark black stool significant for bleeding from upper gastrointestinal tract
Model of End-Stage Liver Disease (MELD): score used to determine placement on the transplant list based on blood test

❧ N

Nutrition: a process of giving the body the key nutrients it needs for proper body function

❧ O

Occupational therapy: therapy that focuses on the activities of daily living such as personal hygiene, bathing, dressing, grooming, toileting, and feeding

Ombudsman: a person who helps residents of a retirement or health care facility with such problems as quality of care, food, finances, medical care, residents rights, and other concerns; these services are confidential and free

Oral hygiene: the process of keeping the mouth clean

❧ P

Passive suicide: killing oneself through indirect action or inaction, such as no longer taking life-prolonging medications

Pathogen: a disease-causing microorganism

Peritoneum: the cavity between intestinal organs and muscle

Peritonitis: infection of the peritoneum

Physical therapy: the process of relearning walking, balancing, and transfers

Portal: relating to the liver

Portal hypertension: high blood pressure in the portal system from cirrhosis

Positioning: placing a person in a position that allows functional activity and minimizes the danger of faulty posture that could cause pressure sores, impaired breathing, and shrinking of muscles and tendons

Power of Attorney for Health Care: providing another person with the authority to make health care decisions

Pressure sore: a breakdown of the skin caused by prolonged pressure in one spot; a bed sore; decubitus ulcer

Prognosis: a forecast of what is likely to happen when an individual contracts a particular disease or condition

Pruritis: generalized itching all over body, can be due to liver disease

❧ Q

Quadriplegia: paralysis of both the upper and lower parts of the body from the neck down

R

Range of motion (ROM): the extent of possible passive (movement by another person) movement in a joint

Rehabilitation: after a disabling injury or disease, restoration of a person's maximum physical, mental, vocational, social, and spiritual potential

Respite care: short-term care that allows a primary caregiver time off from his or her responsibilities

S

Sedatives: medications used to calm a person

Shock: a state of collapse resulting from reduced blood volume and/or blood pressure caused by burns, severe injury, pain, or an emotional blow

Sitz bath: a bath in which only the hips and buttocks are immersed into water or a medicated solution

Spider angiomas: physical finding of small red superficial spots on skin of patient with cirrhosis

Splenomegaly: enlarged spleen, can be due to portal hypertension

Spontaneous bacterial peritonitis: infection in the stomach cavity relating to large amount of ascites

Stroke: sudden loss of function of a part of the brain due to interference in its blood supply, usually by hemorrhage or blood clotting

Support groups: groups of people who get together to share common experiences and help one another cope

Symptom: sign of a disease or disorder that helps in diagnosis

T

Thrombocytopenia: low platelet count

Tracheotomy: surgical procedure to make an opening in a person's windpipe to aid in breathing

Tranquilizers: a class of drugs used to calm a person and control certain emotional disturbances

Transfer: movements from one position to another, for example, from bed to chair, wheelchair to car, etc.

U

Urinal: a container used by a bedridden male for urinating
Urinalysis: a laboratory test of urine

V

Vital signs: life signs such as blood pressure, breathing, and pulse
Void: to urinate; pass water

W

Will: a legal document that states how to dispose of a person's property after death according to that person's wishes

Index

letters of instruction, 75
living trusts, 74
power of attorney, 74
representative payee, 74
Social Security benefits, 80–81
tools, 74
wills, 74
First-aid kit checklist, 212
Food preparation, 187–188
Foreign travel, 171
Funeral expense deductions, 79
Furosemide (Lasix), 42

Generic medications, 41
Grab bars, 96
Ground fault interrupter (GFI), 96
Group Model HMOs, 65
Guilt and caregiver burnout, 119
Gynecomastia, 161

Handwashing, 148–149
Health care team, 33–52
    alternative/complementary treatments, 46
    case management, 50–51
    doctor-patient-caregiver relationship, 36
    doctor selection, 34–35
    health maintenance organizations (HMOs), 34
    hospital stays, 47–50
    mental health treatment, 46–47
    nurse practitioners/physician assistants, 35
    Patient's Bill of Rights during, 47
    preparing for doctor's visit, 36–37
    questions to ask, 40–45
    second opinions, 34, 37
    sharing in medical decisions, 35–40
    watchful waiting option, 37
Health maintenance organizations (HMOs), 34, 65–68
    appealing decisions, 67–68
    complaints, 67
    Group Model, 65
    Individual Practice Associations (Ipsa) plans, 65
    Medicare, 65
    Point of Service (POS) plans, 65

selecting, 65–67
Hemochromatosis, 7
Hemorrhoids, 147
Hepatic encephalopathy, 43, 160, 164
Hepatitis, 6, 14–20
    autoimmune form, AIH, 10
    hepatitis A, 6
    hepatitis B, 6, 14–17
    hepatitis B virus (HBV), 14
    hepatitis C, 6, 17–20
    hepatitis D, 6
    hepatitis E, 6
    hepatitis G, 6
Hepatocellular carcinoma, 25–26
Hepsera. See adefovir
Hereditary liver disease, 5
    alpha-1-antitrypsin deficient (AAT), 8
    hemochromatosis, 7
Home Prepartion, 87–103
    bathroom, 96–97
    bedroom, 100–101
    doorways, 95
    elevators, 94, 95
    kitchen, 98–99
    ramps, 94
    safety, 88–94
    stairways, 90–91, 93
    wheelchair access, 89–90, 94–95
Home first-aid kit checklist, 212
Hospital bed with rails, 101
Hospital stay, 47–50. See also plan of care
    checklist for coming home, 49
    discharge, 48
    ombudsman/advocate, 50
    watching out for patient interests, 47
Hostility and caregiver burnout, 123

Ibuprofen, 9
Income tax issues, 75–80
    charitable giving, 80
    dependent status of care receiver, 55, 76–77
    funeral expense deductions, 79
    gifting, 80
    head of household status, 79
    tax credits for elderly/disabled, 77

Notes

�>➤➤

_____

_____

_____

_____

_____

_____

_____

_____

_____

_____

_____

_____

_____

_____

_____

_____

_____

_____

_____